CONTENTS

1. How to Start Exercise — 1
2. How to get Start — 3
3. Some tips for beginner — 4
4. The health benefits of regular physical exercise — 6
5. Skipping Rope Exercise — 16
6. Cardiovascular Health — 17
7. Decreased Risk of Chronic Diseases — 19
8. Boosted Immune System — 23
9. Increased Muscle Strength — 25
10. Weight Loss — 27
11. Increased Metabolic Rate — 32
12. Aerobic exercise — 33
13. Yoga — 39
14. Better Sleep — 43
15. Progressive Muscle Relaxation — 44
16. Weight lifting — 48
17. Risks of Weight Lifting Exercise — 52
18. Nutrition — 55
19. Nutrition and Disease Prevention — 57
20. Nutrients in Healthy Foods — 62
21. Heart Health — 66
22. Weight Control — 67
23. Improved Brain Health — 68
24. How to Eat Healthy — 69
25. Avoid Processed Foods — 71
26. Fasting — 72

1

How to start exercising and what is the benefit for everyone. Regular exercise is one of the best things for everyone can do for health. you'll begin to see and feel the benefits consistent physical activity can have on your body and well-being quickly. Exercise into your routine takes a lot of determination, and sticking to it in the long term requires discipline. While practical concerns like a busy schedule or poor health can make exercise more challenging, the biggest barriers are mental. May be it's a lack of self-confidence that keeps you from taking positive steps, or your motivation quickly flames out, or you get easily discouraged and give up. We've all been there at some point.

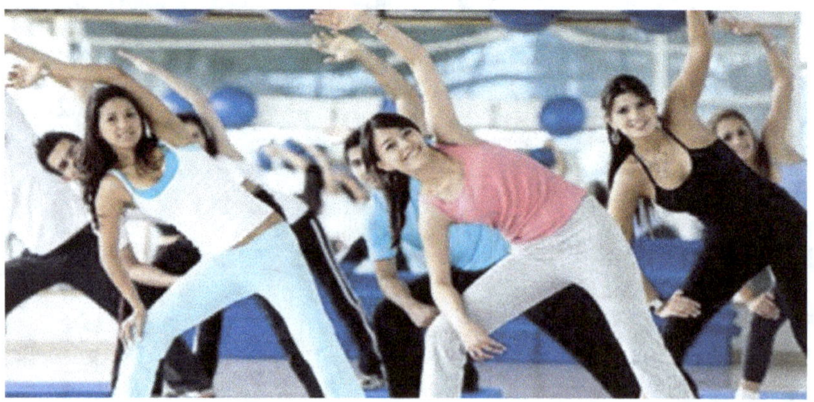

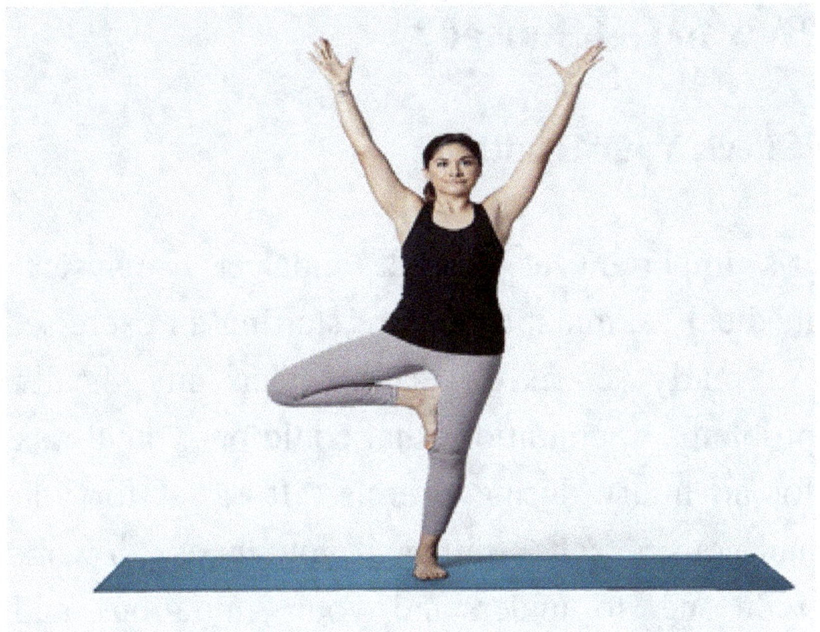

One Question come - Why exercise?

Regular exercise will improve your health significantly and will maintain a healthy body weight and muscle mass and reducing your risk for chronic diseases. It lift your mood, boost your mental health, help you sleep better, and even enhance your sex life. It can also help you maintain good energy levels in short, exercise is powerful and can help improve your life.

3
How to Get Started?

Check Your Health

It's important to consult and get a physical medical examination before starting an exercise. An early check-up can detect any health problems or conditions that could put you at risk for an injury during exercise. It easier for you and your personal trainer, if you choose to work with one, to understand your limitations and create an exercise plan tailored to your particular needs.

We often hear the phrase **"health is wealth"**. While it is true that good health is priceless and invaluable, it can also translate to achieving financial wealth. Many people overlook the fact that a healthy lifestyle not only benefits our physical and mental well-being but can also lead to financial success.

we will explore how to achieve financial riches through a healthy lifestyle.

Some tips for beginners

Warm up:

It's important to warm up before your workout. Doing so can help prevent injuries and improve your athletic performance Simply start your workout with some aerobic exercises like arm swings, leg kicks, and walking.

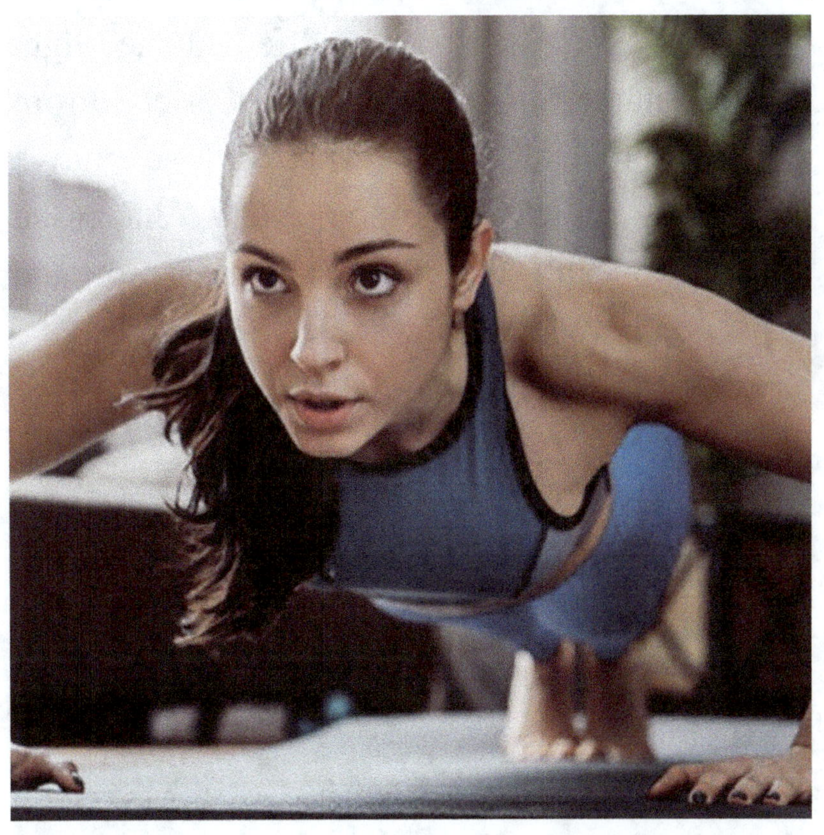

In today's fast-paced and sedentary lifestyle, health and exercise have become crucial elements in maintaining a balanced and fulfilling life. The significance of health and exercise cannot be overstated, as they play a fundamental role in promoting physical, mental, and emotional well-being. This comprehensive essay aims to explore the importance of health and exercise in various aspects of life and shed light on the numerous benefits they offer. From disease prevention to improved cognitive function, enhanced mood, and increased longevity, health and exercise have a profound impact on individuals and society as a whole.

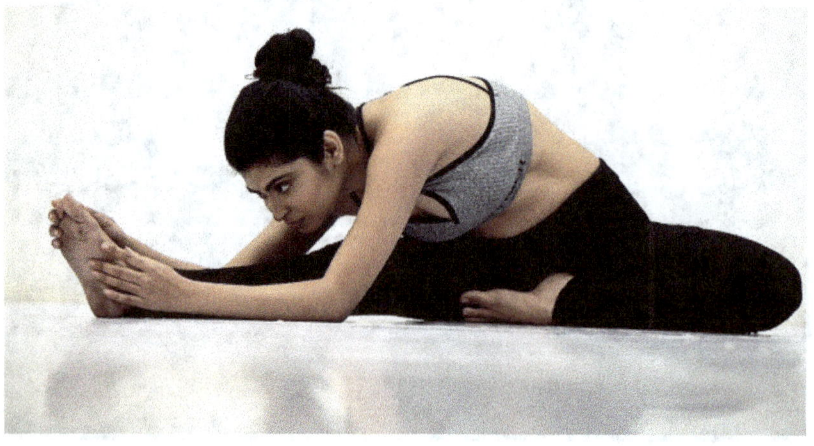

6

The health benefits of regular physical exercise include:

• Weight management and control

• Improved cardiovascular health and reduced risk of heart disease.

• Increased muscle strength, endurance, and flexibility.

• Enhanced bone density and reduced risk of osteoporosis.

• Improved mental health,including reduced stress, anxiety, and depression.

• Enhanced cognitive function and memory.

• Improved sleep quality.

• Reduced risk of chronic diseases such as diabetes, obesity, and certain types of cancer

• Boosted immune system function.

• Improved overall longevity and quality of life.

1.Physical Fitness: Regular exercise helps improve cardiovascular health, increase muscle strength and endurance, enhance flexibility, and maintain a healthy weight. It reduces the risk of chronic diseases such as heart disease, diabetes, obesity, and certain types of cancer.

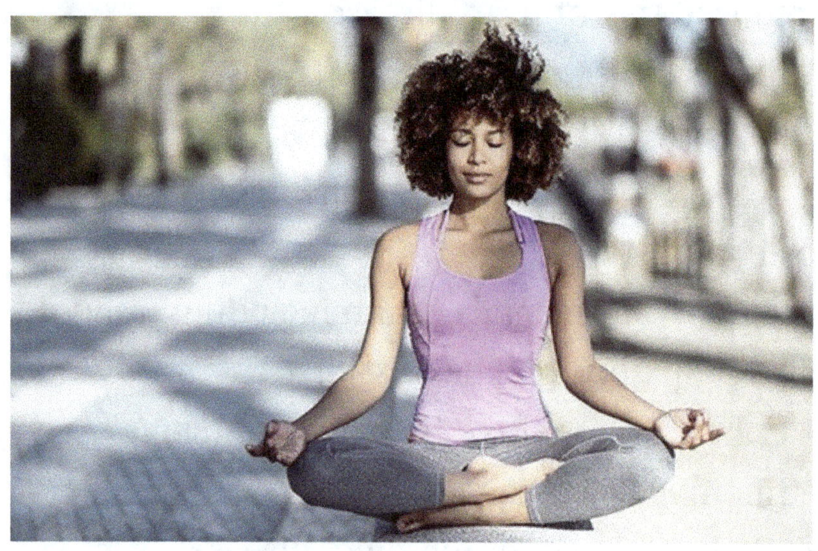

2.Mental Well-being: Engaging in physical activity releases endorphins, which are natural mood boosters that promote feelings of happiness and reduce stress, anxiety, and depression. Exercise also improves cognitive function, memory, and overall mental sharpness.

3. Disease Prevention: A healthy lifestyle that includes exercise and proper nutrition can significantly reduce the risk of various diseases. Regular physical activity strengthens the immune system, improves respiratory function, and lowers the likelihood of developing conditions like osteoporosis, stroke, high blood pressure, and metabolic disorders.

4. Energy and Productivity: Exercise enhances energy levels by improving blood circulation and increasing oxygen supply to the body and brain. Regular physical activity promotes better sleep quality, boosts concentration, enhances productivity, and helps manage daily tasks more effectively.

5. Longevity: Leading an active and healthy lifestyle has been linked to increased life expectancy. Regular exercise, coupled with a balanced diet, can help prevent premature aging, maintain vitality, and improve overall quality of life in the long run.

6. Enhanced Self-Confidence: Engaging in regular exercise and maintaining good health often leads to improved body image and self-esteem. Achieving personal fitness goals, developing physical strength, and feeling good about one's appearance can significantly boost self-confidence and self-worth.

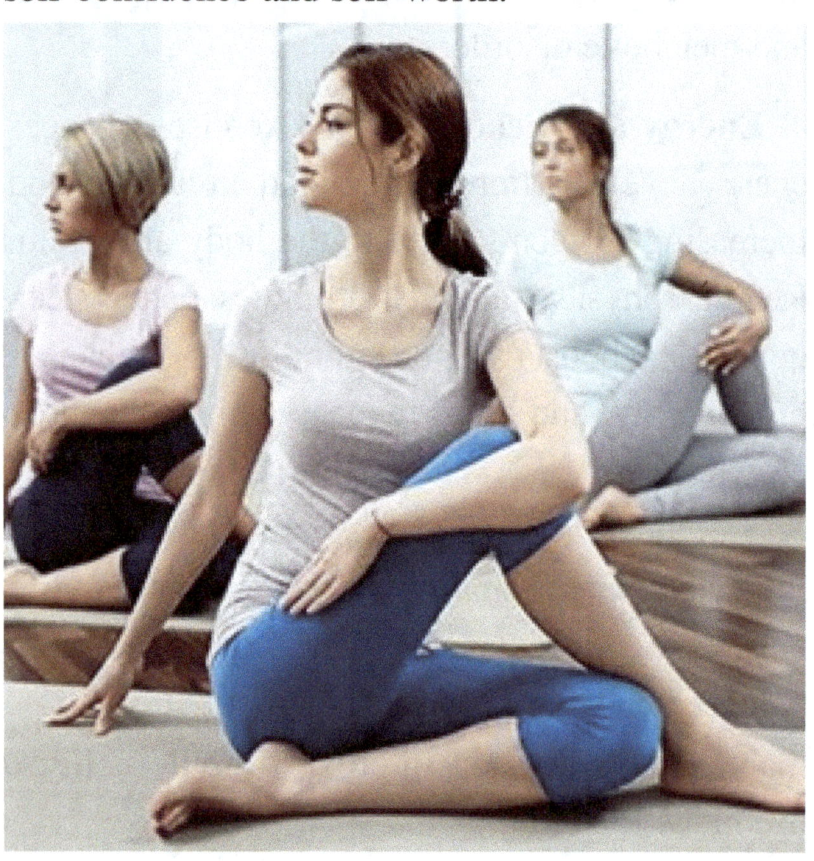

7. Social Connection: Participating in group exercise activities or sports provides opportunities for social interaction and the formation of meaningful relationships. Joining fitness classes, sports teams, or outdoor recreational activities can enhance social well-being, combat loneliness, and promote a sense of belonging.

8. Stress Management: Exercise is an effective way to relieve stress and tension. Physical activity stimulates the production of endorphins, which act as natural stress reducers. Engaging in regular exercise helps clear the mind, improve mood, and provide a healthy outlet for coping with life's challenges.

Remember to consult with a healthcare professional or fitness expert before starting any exercise regimen, especially if you have pre-existing medical conditions or concern.

1. Walking: Walking is a low-impact exercise that helps improve cardiovascular health, strengthens bones and muscles, enhances balance and coordination, and aids in weight management.

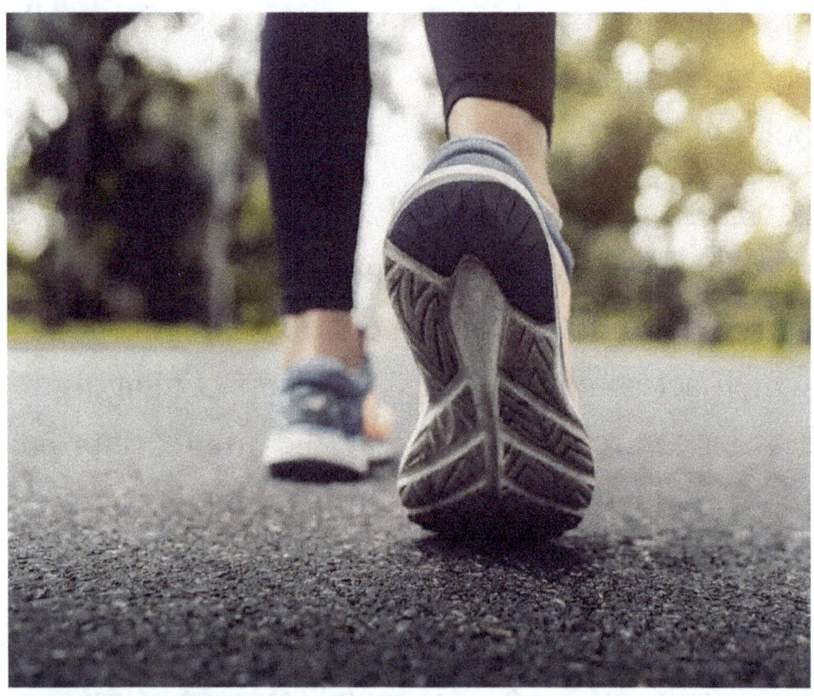

2. Running/Jogging: Running or jogging is an excellent aerobic exercise that boosts cardiovascular fitness, burns calories, improves endurance, strengthens leg muscles, and promotes mental clarity and stress reduction.

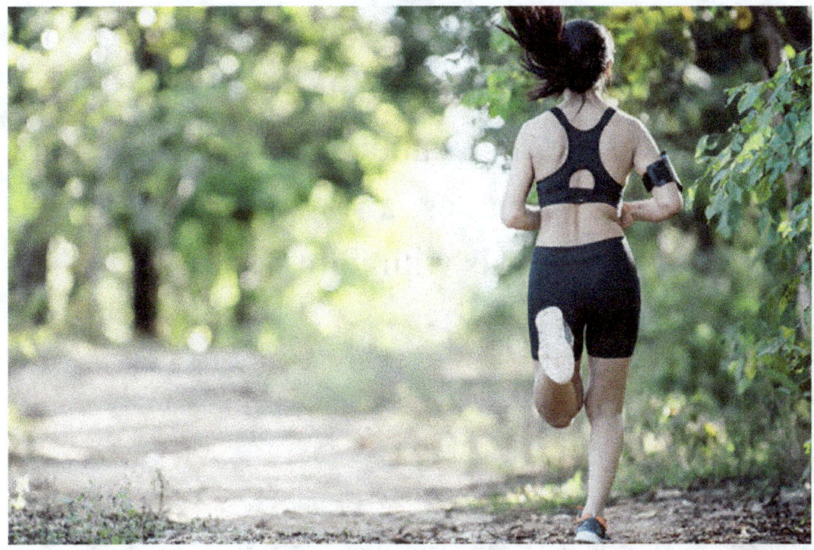

3.Cycling: Cycling is a great cardio-vascular exercise that builds lower body strength, improves joint mobility, increases stamina, and enhances overall cardiovascular health.

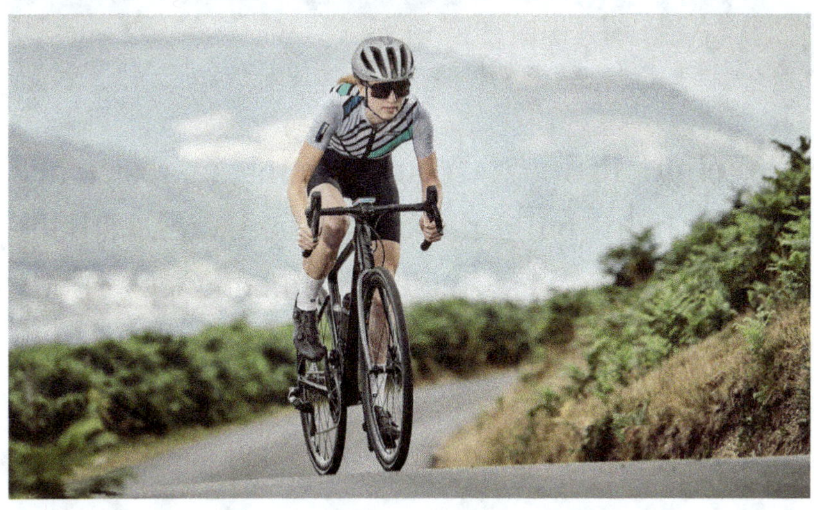

4. Swimming: Swimming is a full-body workout that improves cardiovascular fitness, builds muscle strength and endurance, enhances lung capacity, and provides a low-impact exercise option for individuals with joint issues.

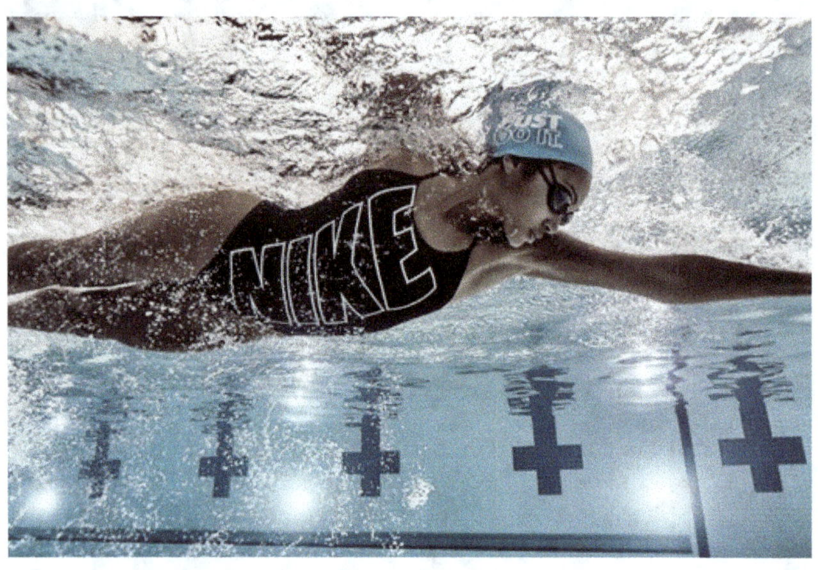

5. Weight lifting : Weight lifting or resistance training helps build muscle mass, increases bone density, improves metabolism,enhances body compo-position, and promotes overall strength and power.

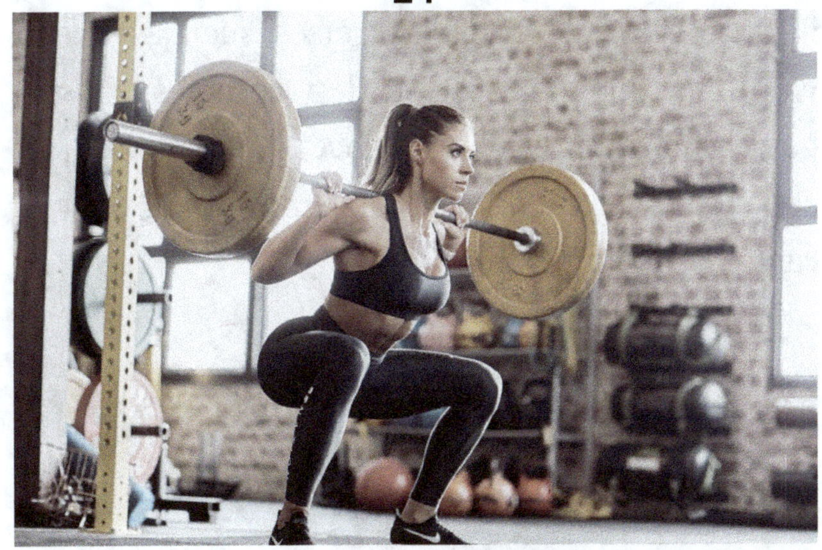

6. Yoga: Yoga combines physical postures, breathing exercises, and meditation to improve flexibility, balance, and strength. It also promotes relaxation, reduces stress, improves mental focus, and enhances overall mind-body connection.

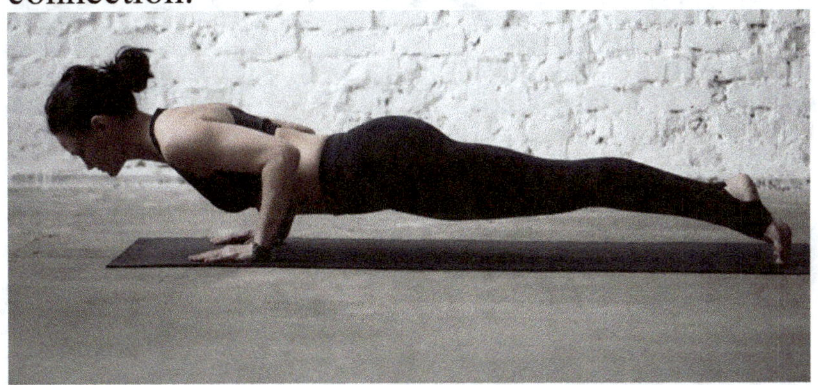

9. Aerobics : Aerobic exercises such as dance workouts, kickboxing, or step aerobics elevate heart rate, improve lung capacity, burn calories, enhance coordination, and promote overall cardiovascular health.

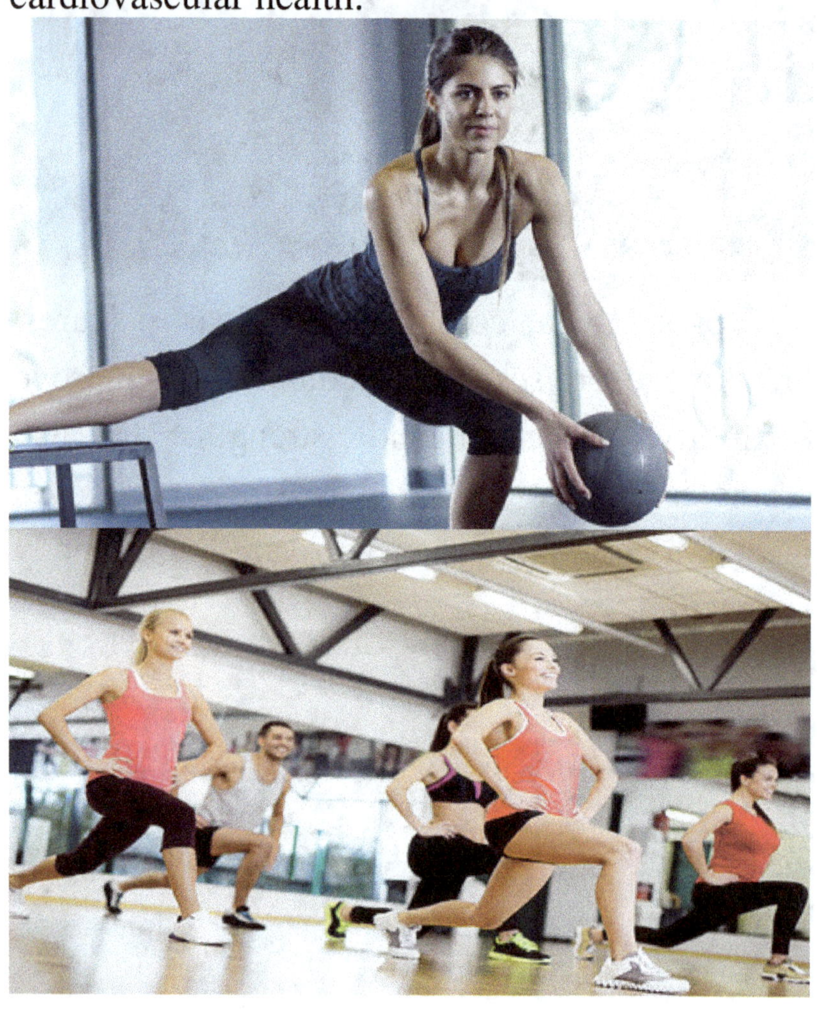

16
Skipping Rope Exercise:

Skipping rope is one of the best exercise for both man and women. There are multiple benefits of skipping rope from losing weight and great calorie-burner. Skipping consistently improves your coordination and stamina. Skipping can help you to improve your stamina. makes your body calm and flexible. Jumping gives great strength to the muscles and relaxes. This can do both indoor and out door.

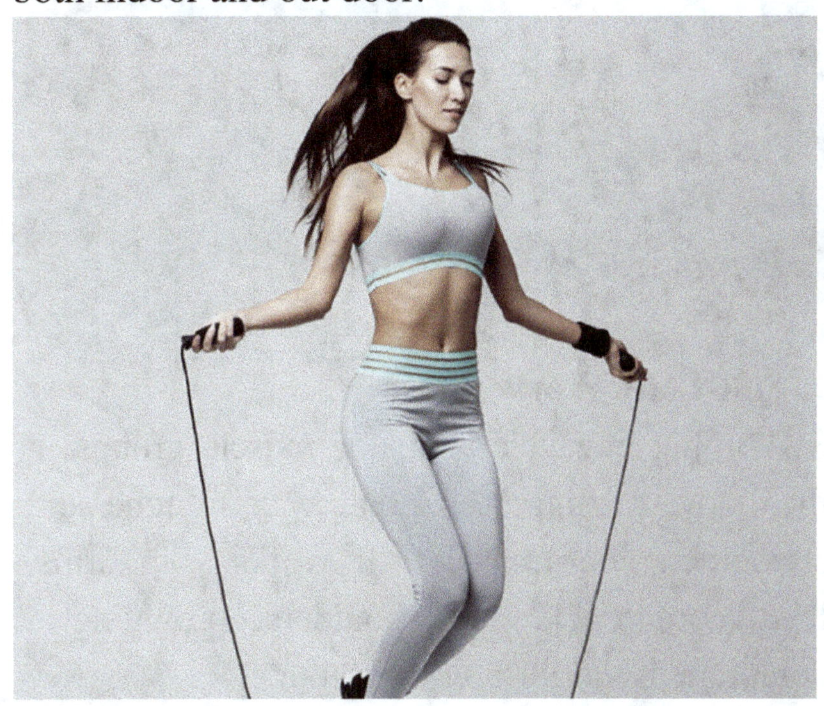

1. Cardiovascular Health:

Swimming is an excellent cardiovascular workout that strengthens the heart and improves its efficiency. It helps lower blood pressure, reduces the risk of heart disease, and improves overall heart health.

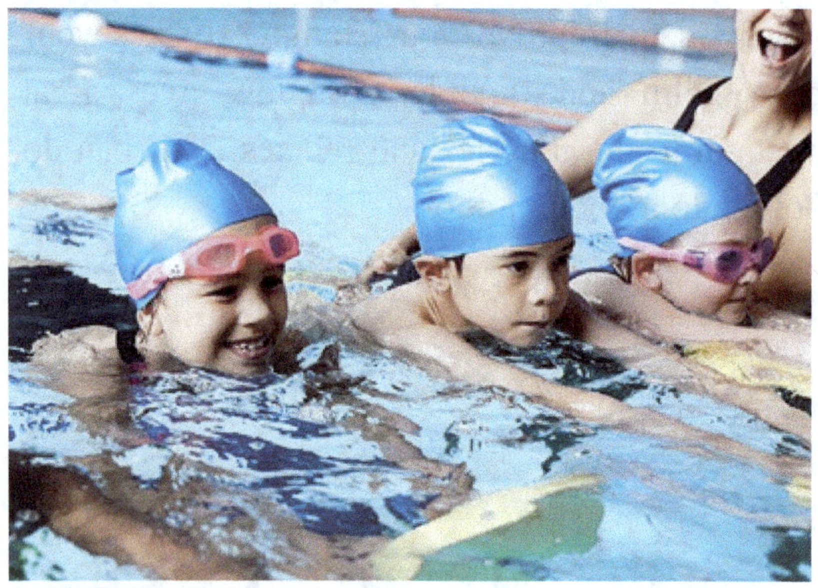

2. Full-Body Workout:

Swimming engages all major muscle groups in the body, making it a great way to tone and strengthen your muscles. It works your arms, legs, core, back, and shoulders, providing a comprehensive full-body workout.

3. Improved Lung Capacity:

Swimming involves controlled breathing techniques, which can improve lung capacity over time. By learning to take deeper, more controlled breaths, swimmers enhance their respiratory muscles and increase their overall lung capacity.

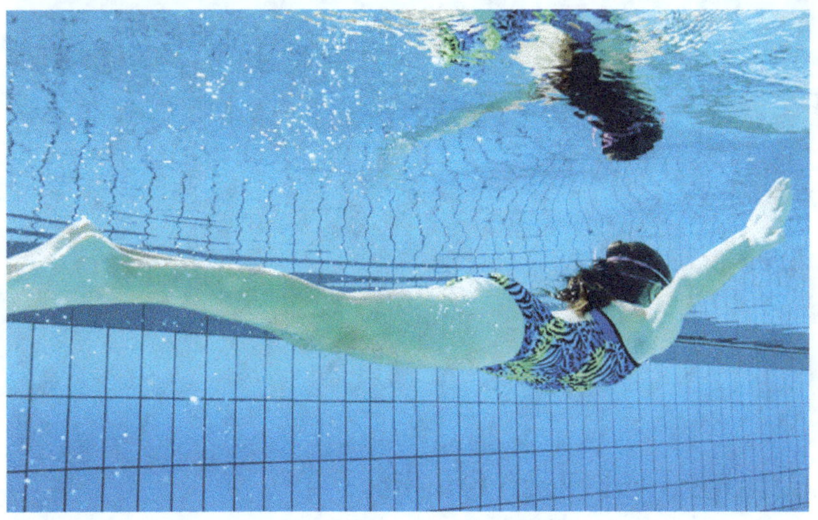

4. Stress Relief:

Swimming has a calming effect on the mind and body. The rhythmic movements and the sensation of being in the water promote relaxation, reduce stress levels, and alleviate anxiety and depression.

5. Decreased Risk of Chronic Diseases:
Engaging in regular swimming can lower the risk of chronic conditions such as type 2 diabetes, stroke, and certain types of cancer. It also helps manage existing conditions like arthritis, asthma, and osteoporosis.

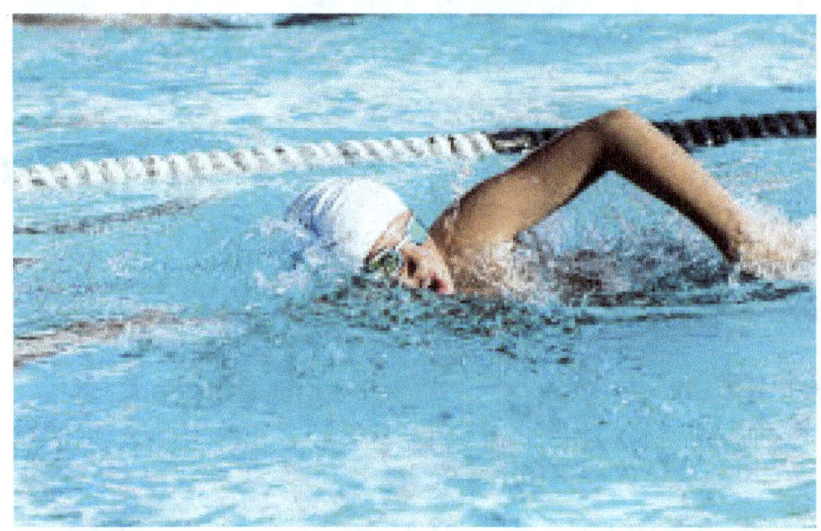

6. Improved Sleep Quality:
Regular physical activity, such as swimming, promotes better sleep patterns. The combination of exercise, relaxation, and the physical fatigue induced by swimming can help you achieve a more restful night's sleep.

1. Cardiovascular Health:

Cycling is a fantastic aerobic exercise that gets your heart pumping and increases blood circulation. Regular cycling helps strengthen the heart, lowers resting heart rate, reduces the risk of heart disease, and improves overall cardiovascular fitness.

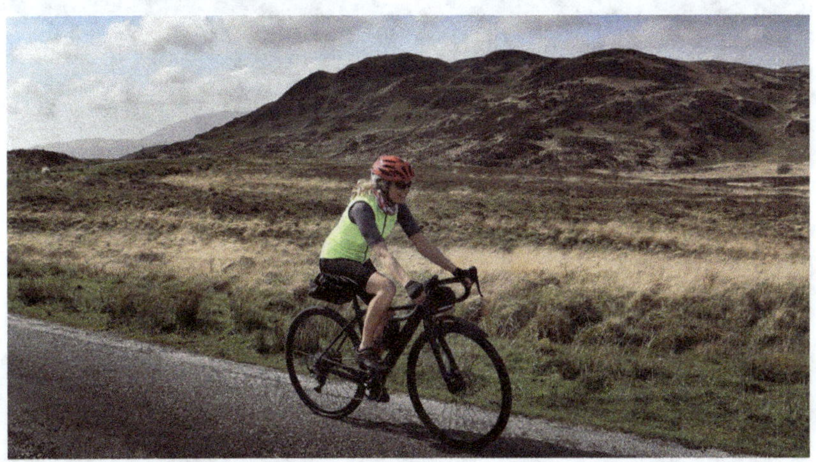

2. Weight Management:

Cycling is an effective way to burn calories, making it an excellent activity for weight management. A moderate-intensity cycling session can burn around 300-600 calories per hour, depending on factors like speed, terrain, and body weight.

3. Muscle Strength and Tone:

Cycling primarily engages the muscles in the legs, including the quadriceps, hamstrings, calves, and glutes. Regular cycling helps strengthen and tone these muscles, resulting in improved lower body strength and endurance.

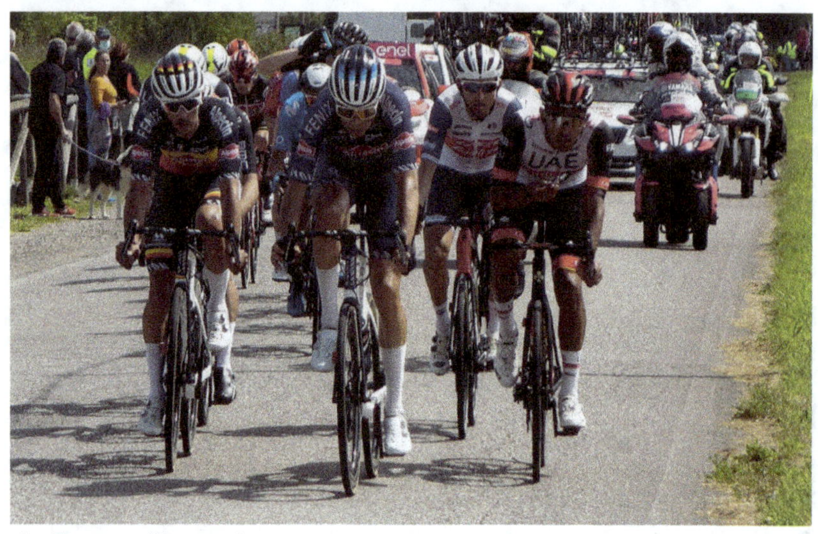

4. Bone Density:

Cycling is a weight-bearing exercise that places stress on the bones, which helps stimulate the growth and maintenance of bone tissue. Regular cycling can contribute to the development of strong bones and reduce the risk of osteoporosis and fractures.

5. Improved Lung Function:

Engaging in regular cycling can help improve lung capacity and function. As cycling requires deep and controlled breathing, it helps strengthen the respiratory muscles and enhances overall lung health.

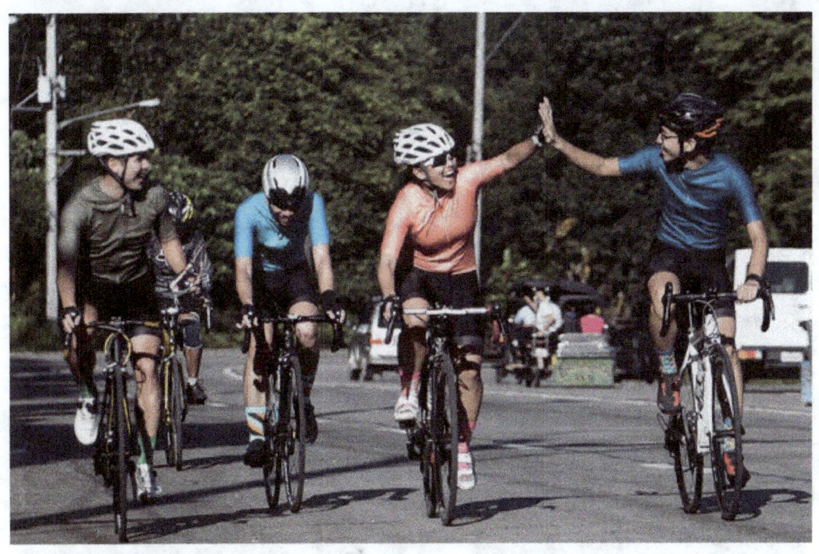

6. Increased Energy Levels:

Cycling is an excellent way to boost energy levels and combat fatigue. Regular exercise improves the delivery of oxygen and nutrients to the body's tissues, enhancing overall energy production and stamina.

1. Boosted Immune System:

Moderate-intensity running strengthens the immune system, reducing the frequency and severity of illnesses like the common cold and flu.

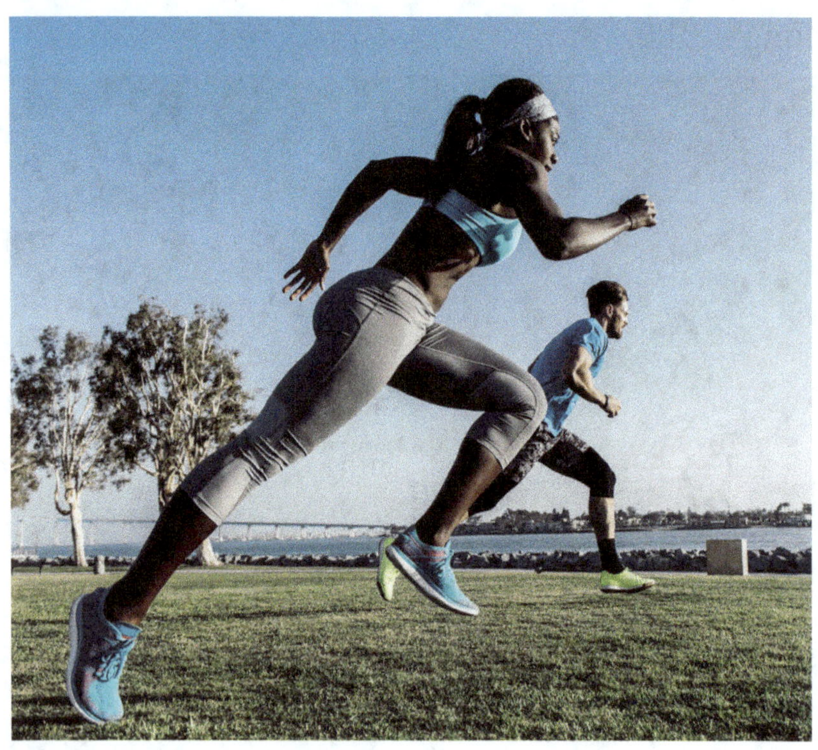

2. Improved cardiovascular health:

Running helps strengthen your heart and improves blood circulation, reducing the risk of heart disease, high blood pressure, and stroke.

3. Increased Lung Capacity:

Running improves lung function, enhances oxygen intake, and strengthens the respiratory system, benefiting overall lung health.

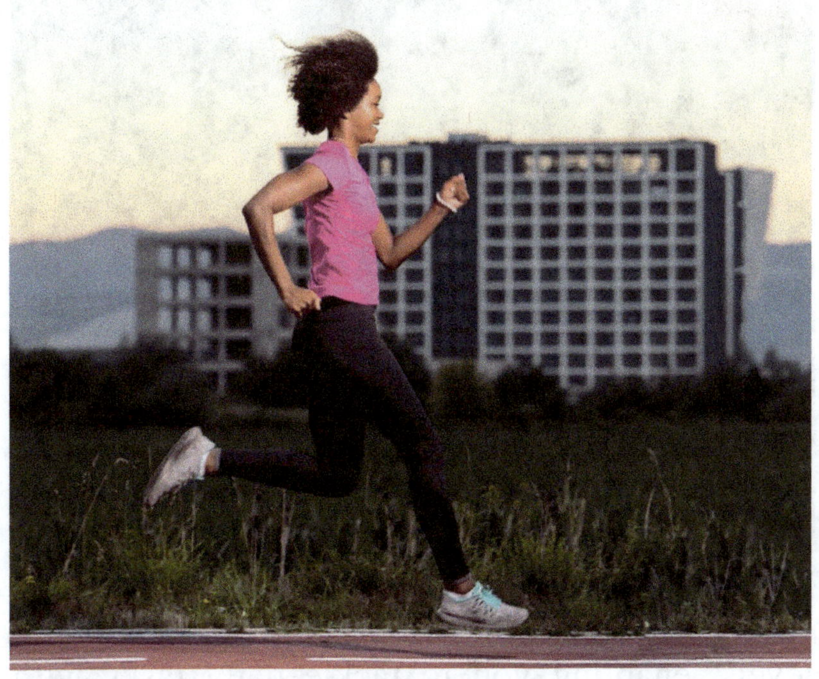

4. Enhanced mental well-being:

Running stimulates the release of endorphins, known as "feel-good" hormones, which can alleviate stress, anxiety, and depression, promoting mental well-being.

5. Increased Muscle Strength:

Running engages multiple muscle groups, especially in the lower body, leading to improved muscle tone, strength, and endurance.

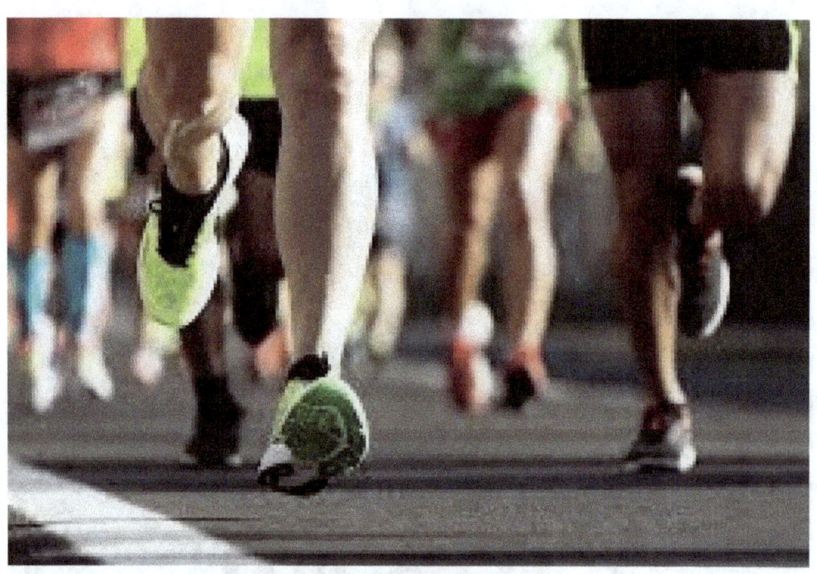

7. Increased Energy Levels:

Running regularly improves stamina and energy levels, enabling you to tackle daily tasks with greater vitality.

8. Stress Relief:

Running serves as a natural stress reliever, helping to clear the mind, improve mood, and reduce tension.

9. Increased Social Connections:

Joining a running club or participating in group runs can provide opportunities to meet like-minded individuals and develop new friendships.

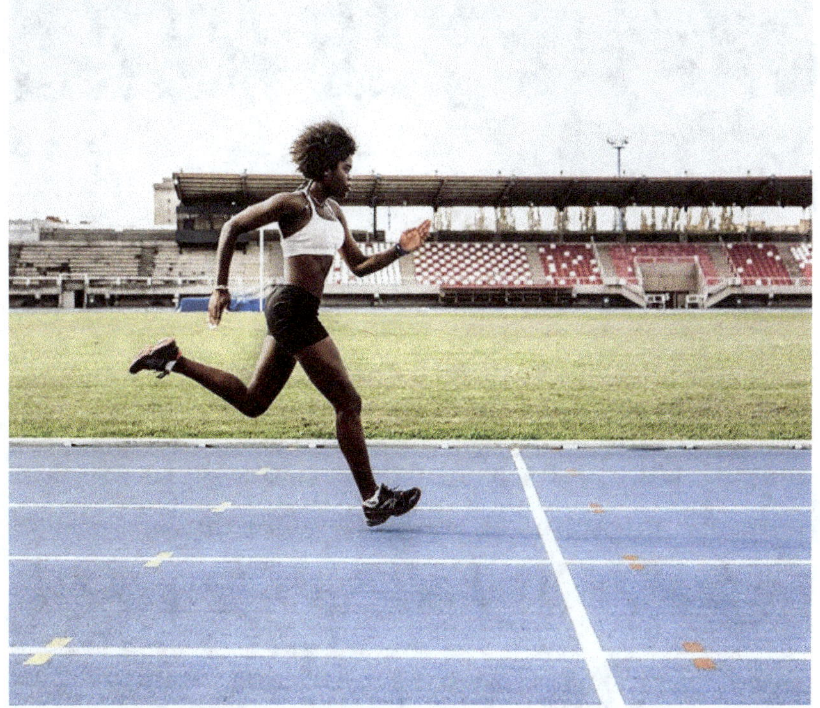

10. Better Balance and Coordination:

Running requires good balance and coordination, and regular practice can enhance these skills, reducing the risk of falls and improving overall physical performance.

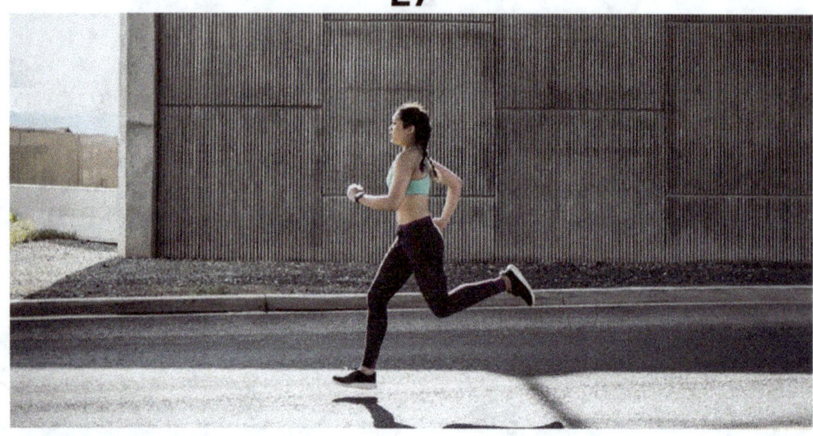

1.Weight Loss: Skipping is a highly effective exercise for weight loss. It burns a significant number of calories in a short amount of time, making it an efficient way to shed excess pounds. Incorporating skipping into your routine can contribute to a calorie deficit, helping you achieve and maintain a healthy weight.

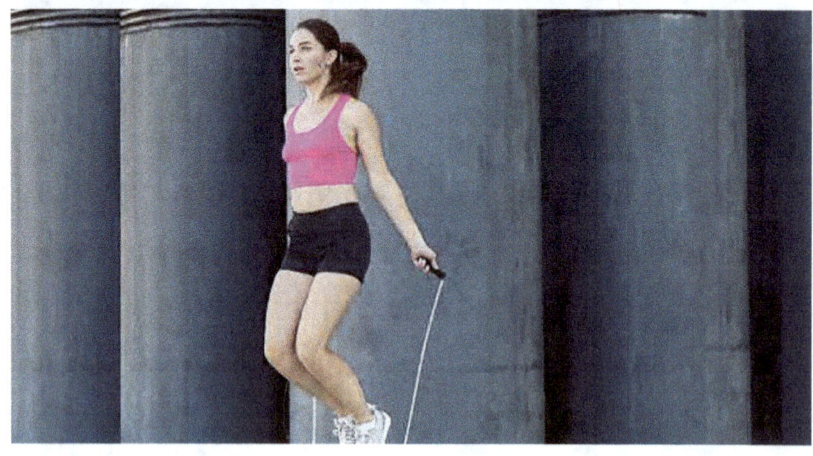

2. Muscle Tone: Skipping engages multiple muscle groups, including the legs, arms, shoulders, and core. Regular skipping sessions can help tone and strengthen these muscles, leading to improved muscle definition and overall body composition

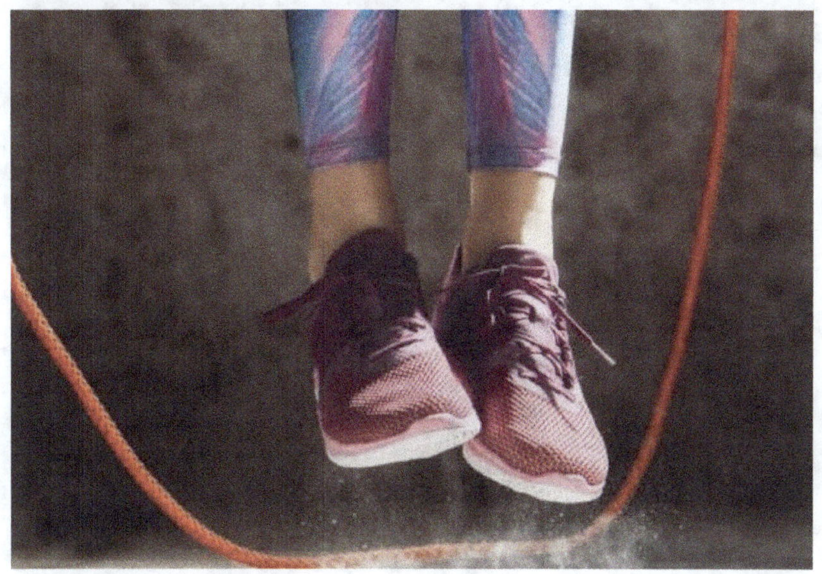

3. Bone Strength: Jumping rope is a weight-bearing exercise, which means it puts stress on your bones. This stress stimulates bone growth and helps increase bone density, reducing the risk of osteoporosis and improving overall bone health.

4. Balance and Coordination: Skipping requires coordination and balance as you time your jumps and maintain a steady rhythm. Regular practice can improve these skills, enhancing your overall balance, agility, and motor coordination.

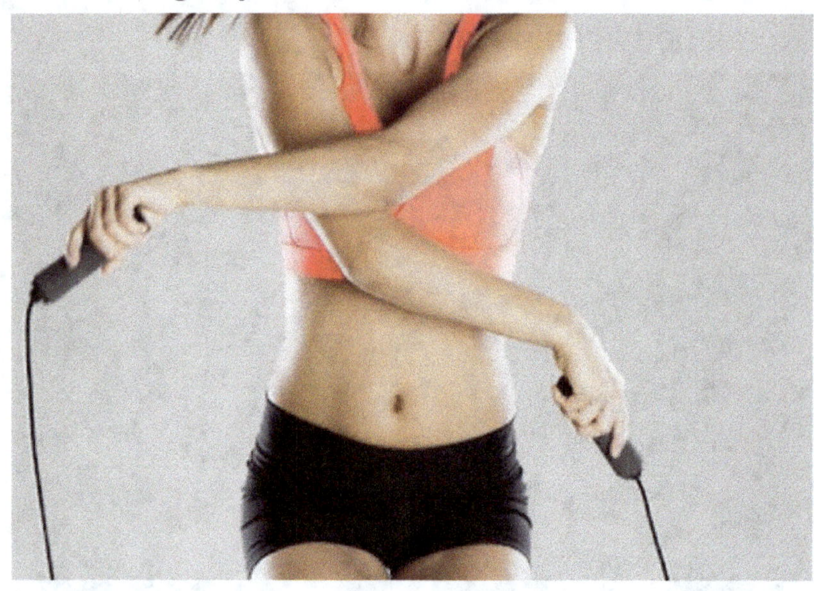

5. Fun and Versatile: Skipping is a fun and versatile exercise that can be tailored to your fitness level and preferences. You can experiment with different skipping techniques, speed variations, and incorporate other exercises, such as high knees or double unders, to add variety and challenge to your workouts.

6. Portable and Affordable: One of the great advantages of skipping is its portability and affordability. You can skip rope virtually anywhere, making it a convenient exercise option. Additionally, jump ropes are relatively inexpensive and require minimal equipment.

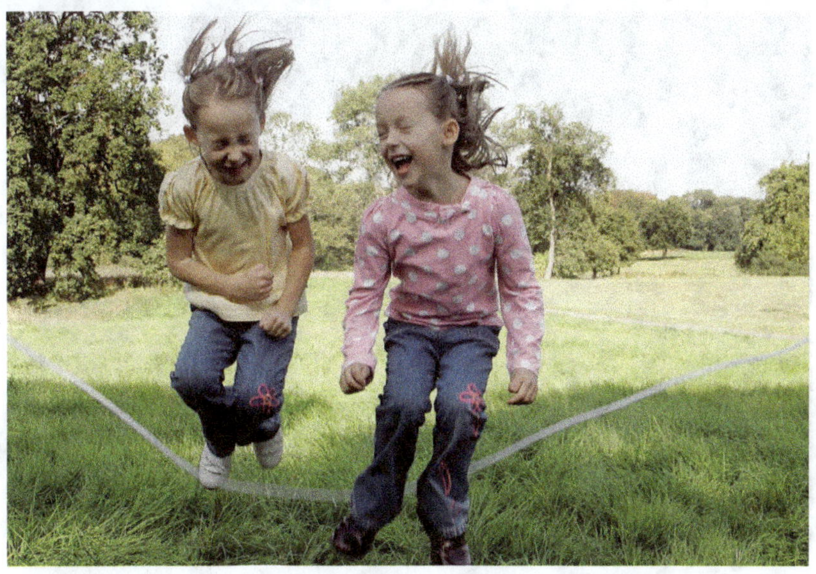

7. Improved Lung Function: Skipping is an aerobic exercise that requires deep and controlled breathing. This helps expand lung capacity, enhances oxygen uptake, and strengthens respiratory muscles, leading to improved lung function and better overall respiratory health.

8. Enhanced Flexibility: The continuous jumping and footwork involved in skipping can improve your flexibility over time. Regular skipping sessions help loosen tight muscles, increase joint mobility, and enhance overall flexibility.

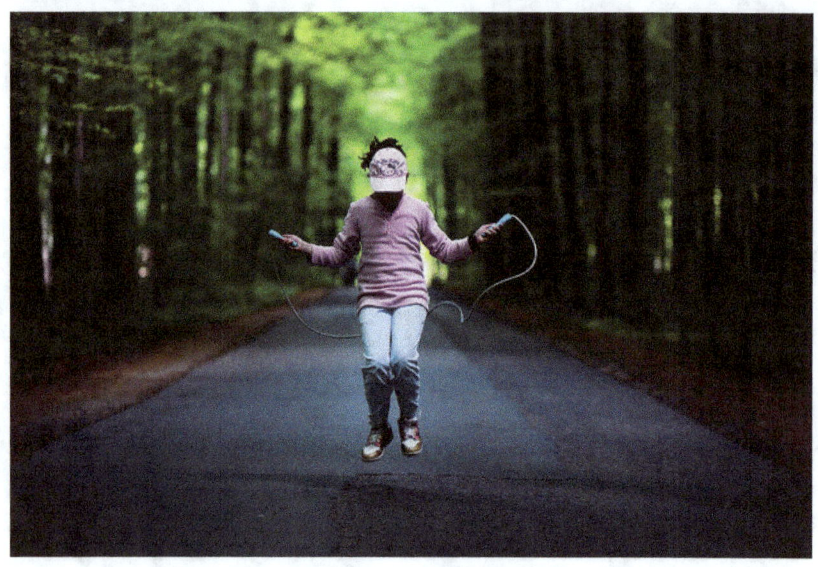

9. Increased Energy Levels: Engaging in regular skipping sessions can boost your energy levels and combat feelings of fatigue. The combination of physical activity, increased blood flow, and the release of endorphins can leave you feeling more energized and rejuvenated.

10. Increased Metabolic Rate: Skipping elevates your heart rate and boosts your metabolism. This increase in metabolic rate can lead to improved calorie burning even after you've finished your workout, contributing to weight loss and weight management.

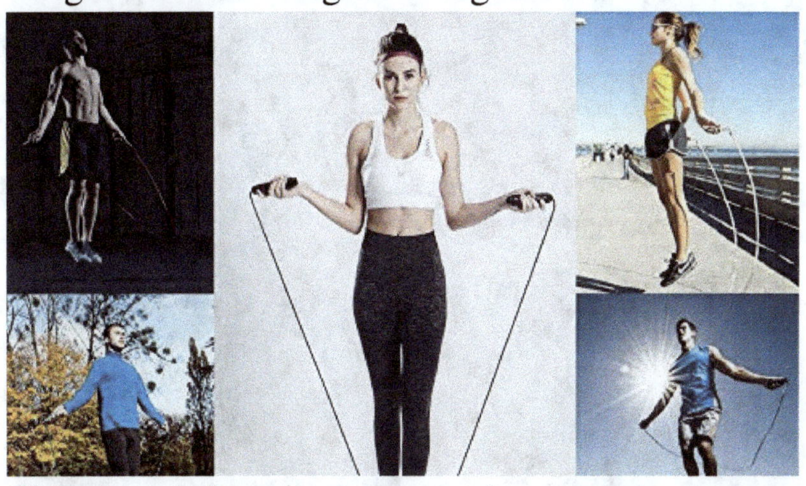

Skipping, also known as jump rope, is an incredibly effective and versatile exercise that can provide a wide range of health benefits. Whether you're a child rediscovering the joy of skipping rope or an adult incorporating it into your fitness routine, the benefits are plentiful. From cardiovascular health to coordination and weight management,

Aerobic exercise, also known as cardio exercise, is a form of physical activity that increases your heart rate and breathing for an extended period. Engaging in regular aerobic exercise has numerous health benefits, both for your physical and mental well-being.

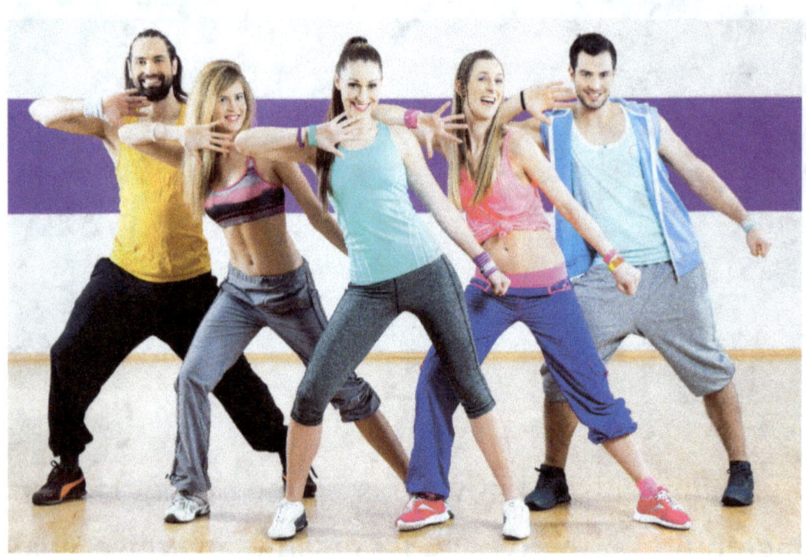

1. Weight Management: Regular aerobic exercise can help you maintain a healthy weight or lose weight if you have excess body fat. It burns calories, boosts metabolism, and contributes to a negative energy balance, leading to weight loss and improved body composition.

2. Increased Lung Capacity: Aerobic exercise challenges your respiratory system, enhancing lung capacity and oxygen uptake. This leads to improved endurance and better overall respiratory function.

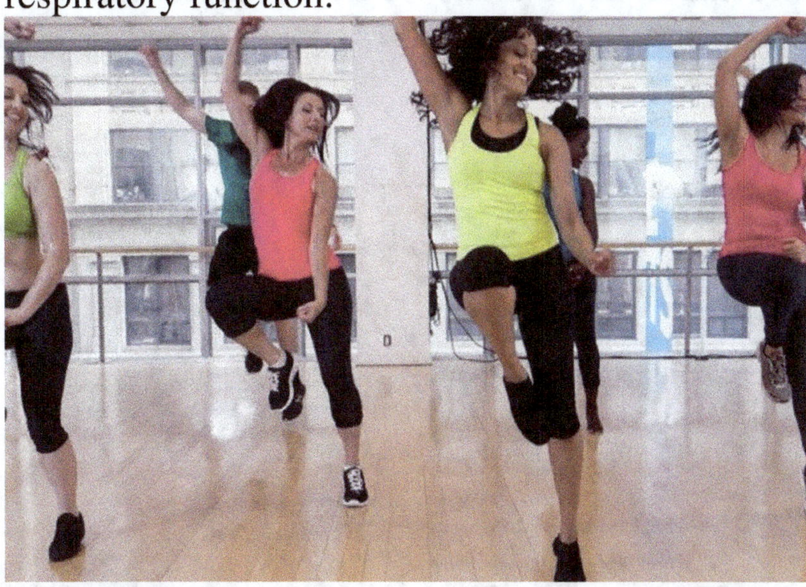

3. Enhanced Mood and Mental Health: Engaging in aerobic exercise triggers the release of endorphins, known as "feel-good" hormones, which promote feelings of happiness and well-being. It can help alleviate symptoms of depression, anxiety, and stress, while improving overall mood and mental health.

4. Stronger Immune System: Consistent aerobic exercise has been shown to strengthen the immune system and reduce the risk of developing chronic diseases. It improves the circulation of immune cells, enhances antibody response, and lowers the risk of infections and illnesses.

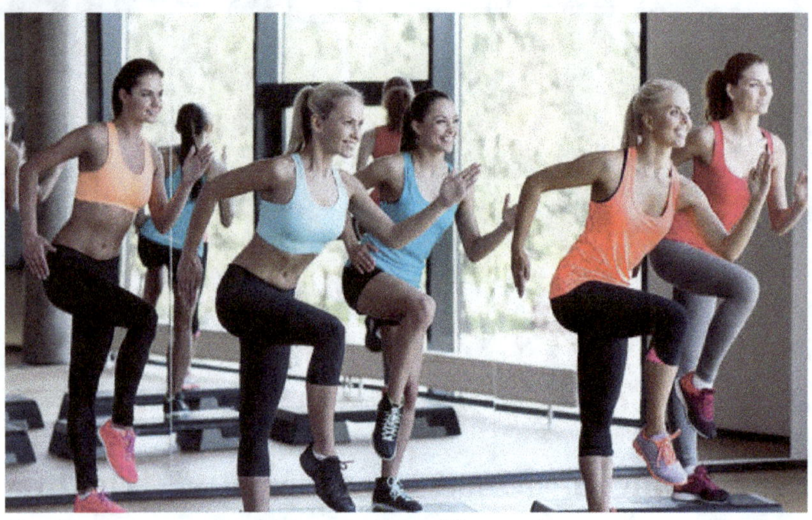

5. Improved Sleep Quality: Regular aerobic exercise can help regulate your sleep patterns, making it easier to fall asleep and improving the overall quality of your sleep. It can reduce insomnia, promote deeper sleep, and enhance daytime alertness.

6. Improved Insulin Sensitivity: Aerobic exercise increases insulin sensitivity, allowing your cells to better utilize glucose and maintain stable blood sugar levels. This is particularly beneficial for individuals with insulin resistance or type 2 diabetes.

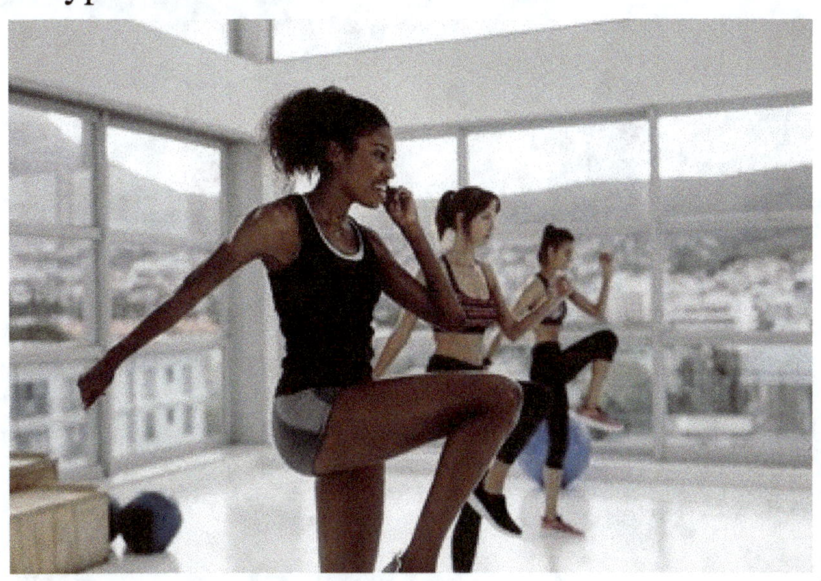

7. Reduced Inflammation:

Chronic inflammation is associated with various health problems, including heart disease, diabetes, and arthritis. Aerobic exercise has anti-inflammatory effects, reducing systemic inflammation and promoting overall health.

8. Reduced Risk of Chronic Diseases: Engaging in aerobic exercise on a regular basis can lower the risk of developing various chronic conditions, including type 2 diabetes, certain types of cancer, stroke, and metabolic syndrome.

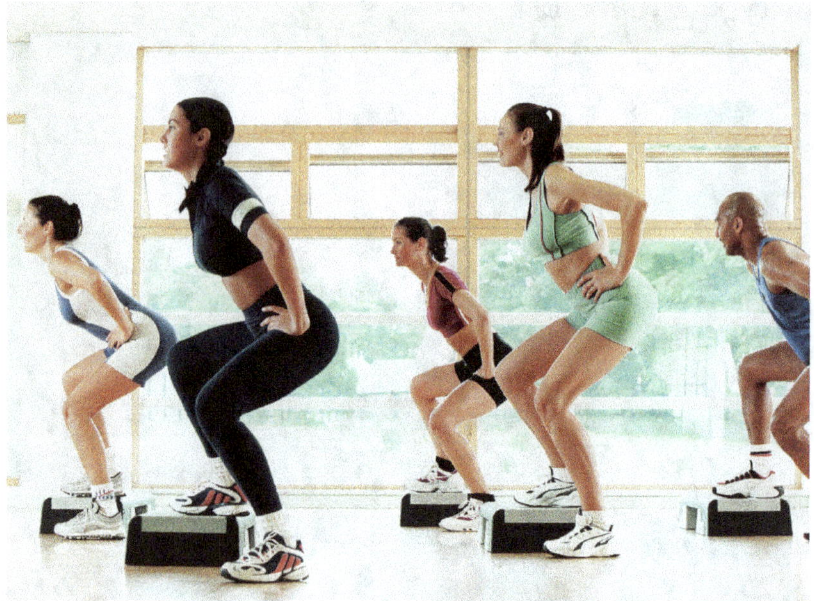

9. Enhanced Longevity: Regularly engaging in aerobic exercise has been linked to increased life expectancy and a reduced risk of premature death. It promotes overall health, helps maintain a healthy weight, and reduces the risk of chronic diseases associated with premature mortality.

10. Social Benefits: Participating in aerobic exercise, such as group fitness classes or team sports, provides social interaction and opportunities for building connections with others who share similar interests. This can improve social well-being and overall happiness.

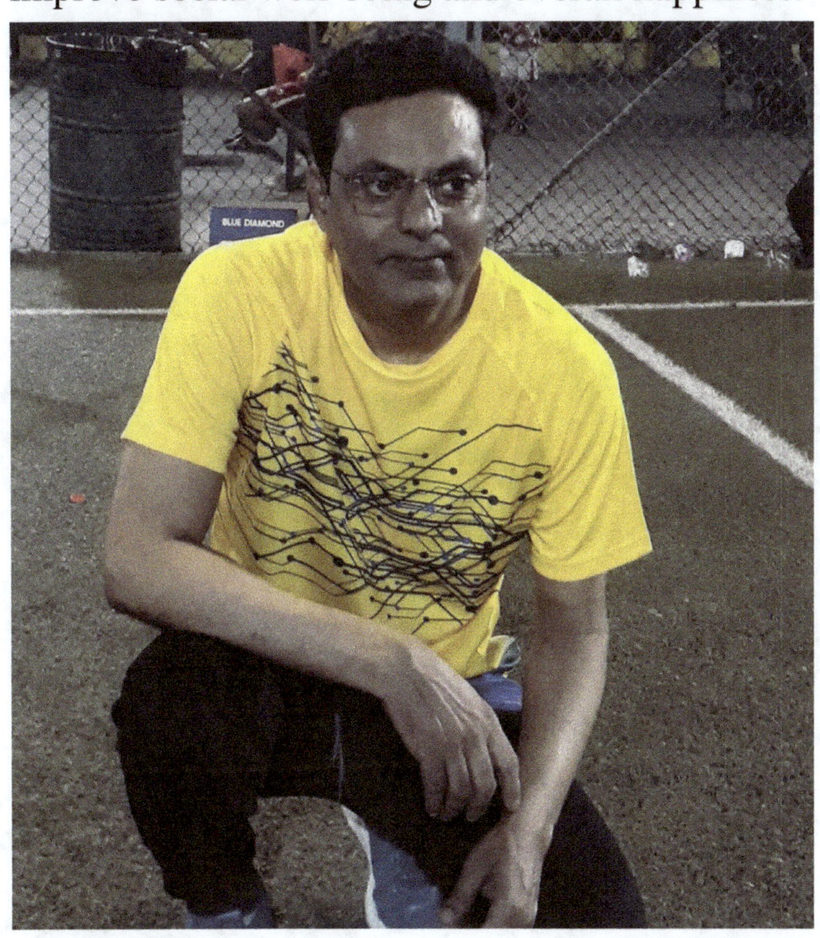

Yoga is a centuries-old practice that encompasses physical postures, breathing exercises, meditation, and ethical principles. It offers numerous benefits for both the body and mind.

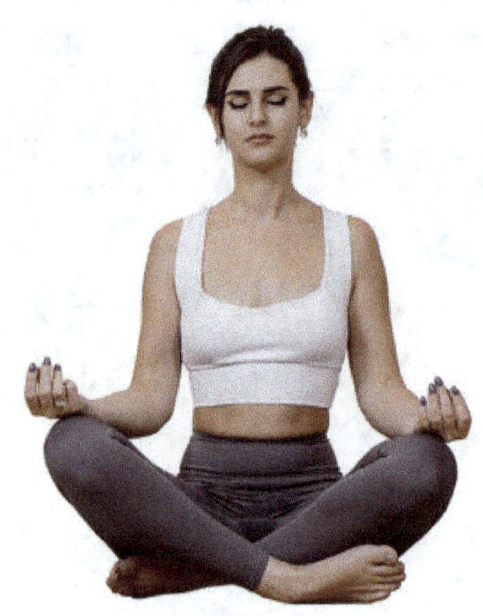

1. Improved Posture: Many yoga poses focus on proper alignment, which helps improve posture. By strengthening the core muscles and aligning the spine, yoga contributes to better posture and reduces the risk of back and neck pain.

2. Physical Fitness: Regular yoga practice improves flexibility, strength, and balance. It helps tone muscles, increases endurance, and enhances overall physical fitness.

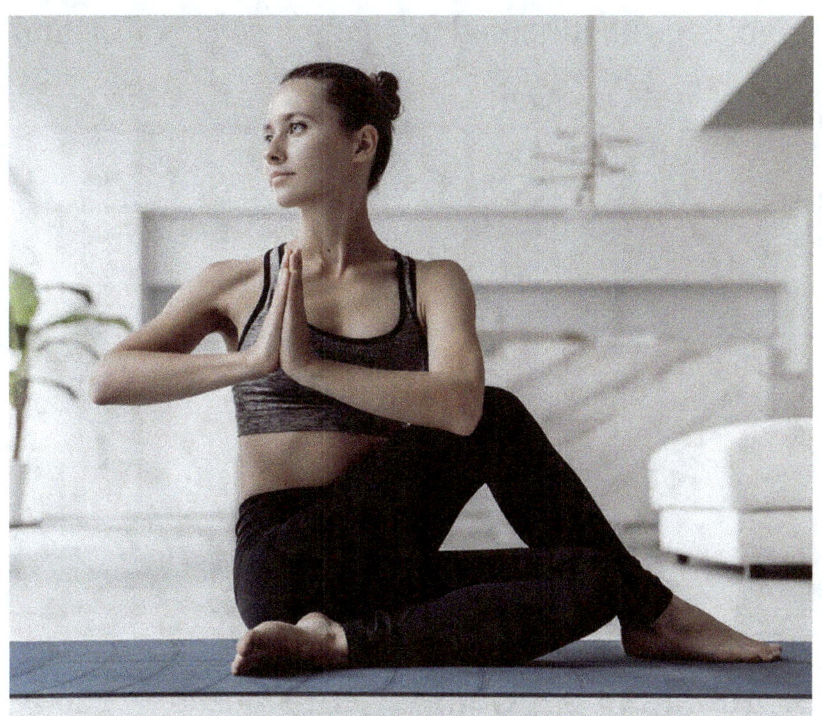

3. Stress Reduction:

Yoga incorporates relaxation techniques such as deep breathing and meditation, which help calm the mind and reduce stress levels. It promotes a sense of inner peace and tranquility.

4. Mental Clarity and Focus: The combination of physical movement, breath control, and meditation in yoga helps enhance mental clarity and concentration. Regular practice can improve cognitive function and promote a sense of mental well-being.

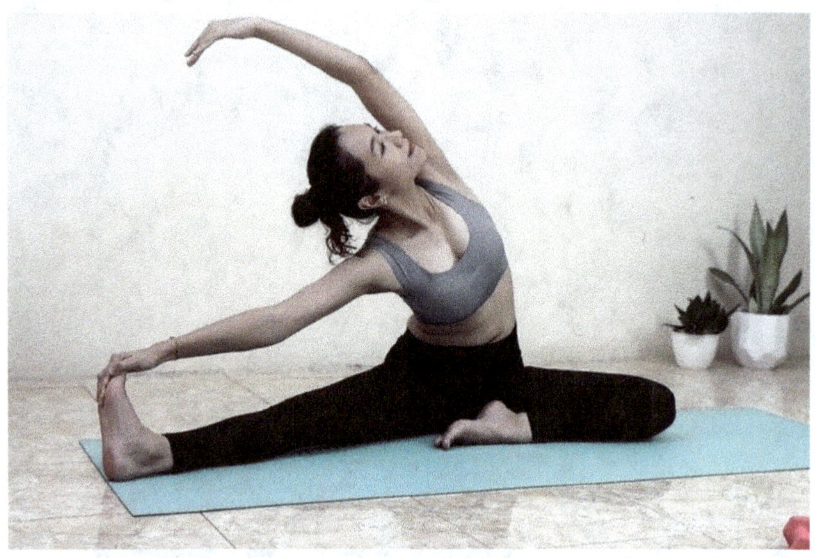

5. Enhanced Flexibility: Yoga postures gently stretch and lengthen muscles, tendons, and ligaments, increasing overall flexibility. Improved flexibility not only supports better physical performance but also helps prevent injuries.

6. Emotional Balance:

Yoga helps create a balance between the body and mind, enabling individuals to connect with their emotions more effectively. It cultivates self-awareness and emotional resilience, leading to improved emotional well-being.

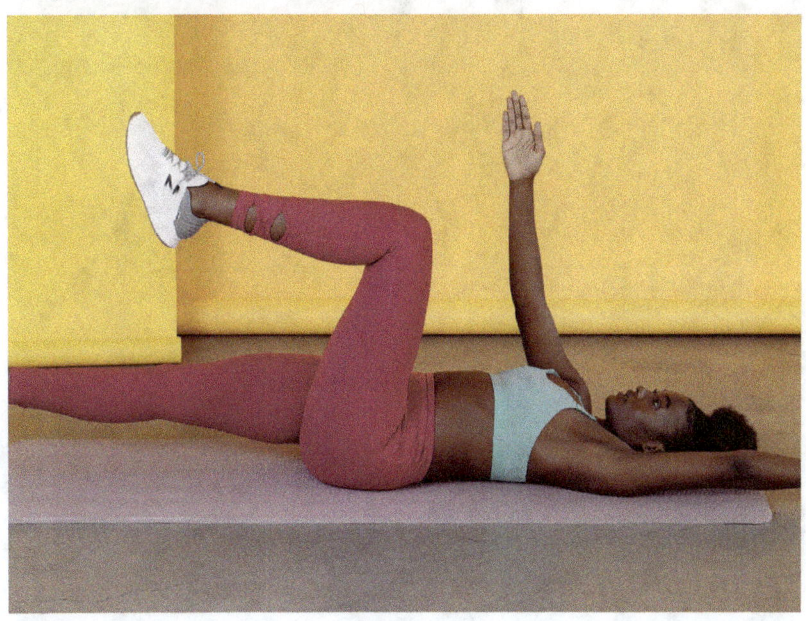

7. Stress Management: Yoga provides effective tools for managing stress. Breathing exercises and meditation techniques can be utilized during challenging situations to induce a state of calmness and reduce stress levels.

8. Better Sleep:

The relaxation techniques practiced in yoga can help combat insomnia and improve the quality of sleep. Yoga also promotes relaxation and reduces anxiety, allowing for a more restful night's sleep.

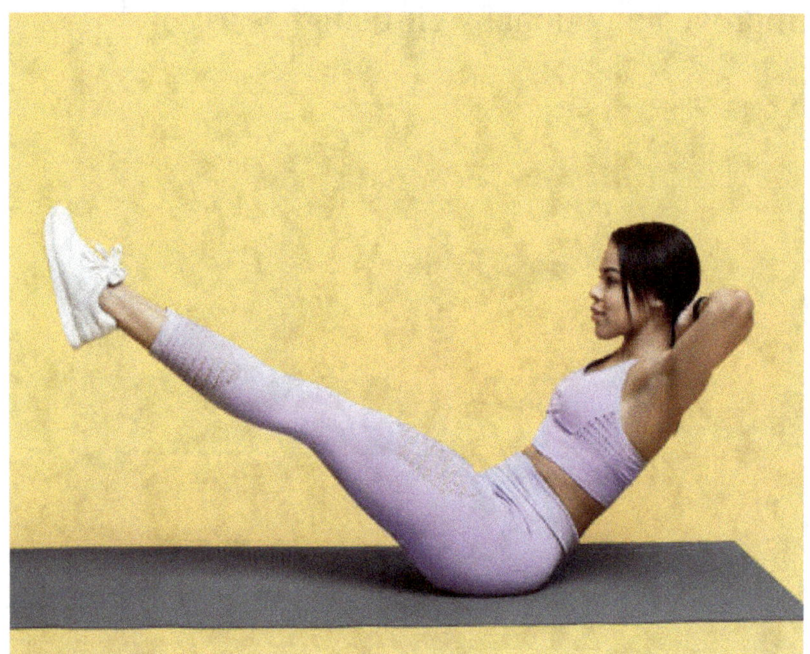

9. Increased Energy Levels: Yoga stimulates the body's energy systems, promoting the flow of vital energy (prana). This leads to increased vitality and improved energy levels throughout the day.

Progressive Muscle Relaxation (PMR) is a relaxation technique that involves tensing and releasing different muscle groups in your body to promote deep relaxation and relieve mental stress. Follow these steps for a guided PMR exercise:

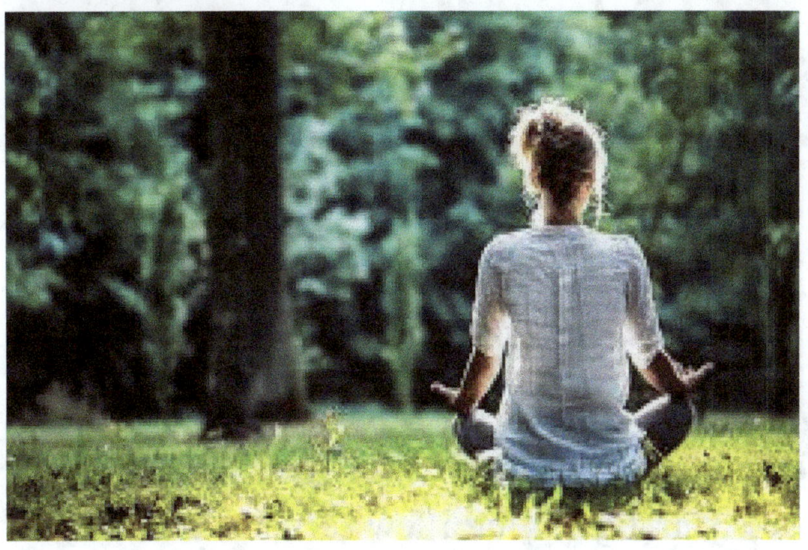

1. Find a quiet and comfortable space where you can relax without interruptions.

2. Sit or lie down in a relaxed position. Close your eyes and take a few deep breaths to center yourself.

3. Start by focusing on your breathing. Inhale slowly through your nose, hold for a few seconds, and exhale through your mouth. Repeat this a few times to calm your mind.

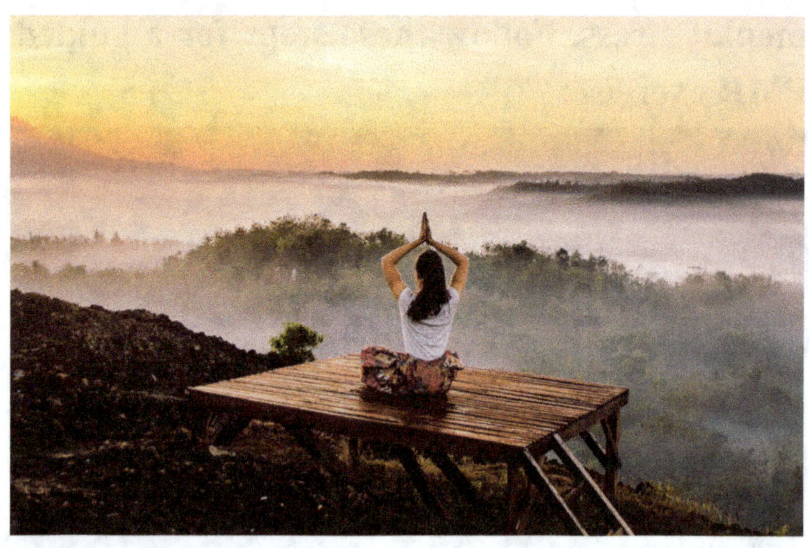

4. Begin with your facial muscles. Squeeze your eyes shut tightly for a few seconds, then release and let the tension go. Allow your facial muscles to relax completely.

5. Move down to your neck and shoulders. Raise your shoulders up towards your ears, hold the tension, and then release, letting them drop and relax. Feel the tension melting away.

6. Proceed to your arms and hands. Clench your fists tightly, hold for a few seconds, and then release. Feel the warmth and relaxation spread through your arms and hands.

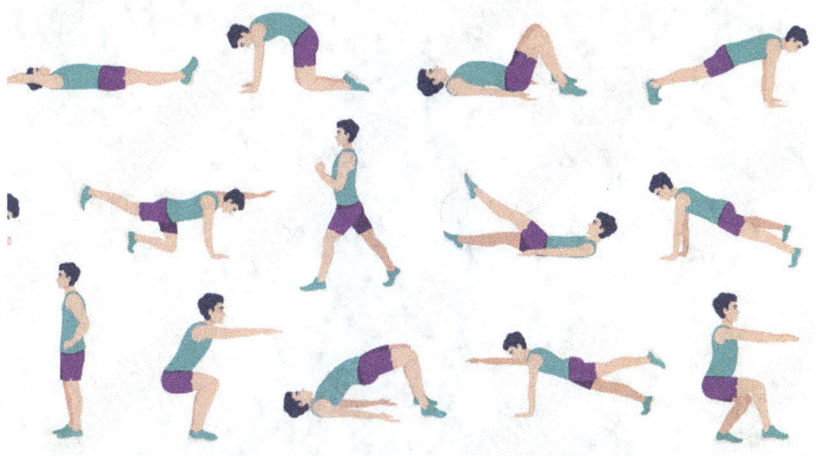

7. Focus on your chest and abdomen. Take a deep breath, expanding your chest and stomach, and then exhale slowly, releasing any tension you feel in these areas.

8. Move to your back and torso. Arch your back slightly, creating tension, and then release and relax. Feel the weight of your body sinking into the surface beneath you.

9. Direct your attention to your legs and feet. Tense your leg muscles by pointing your toes towards your face, hold for a few seconds, and then release. Feel the heaviness and relaxation in your legs and feet.

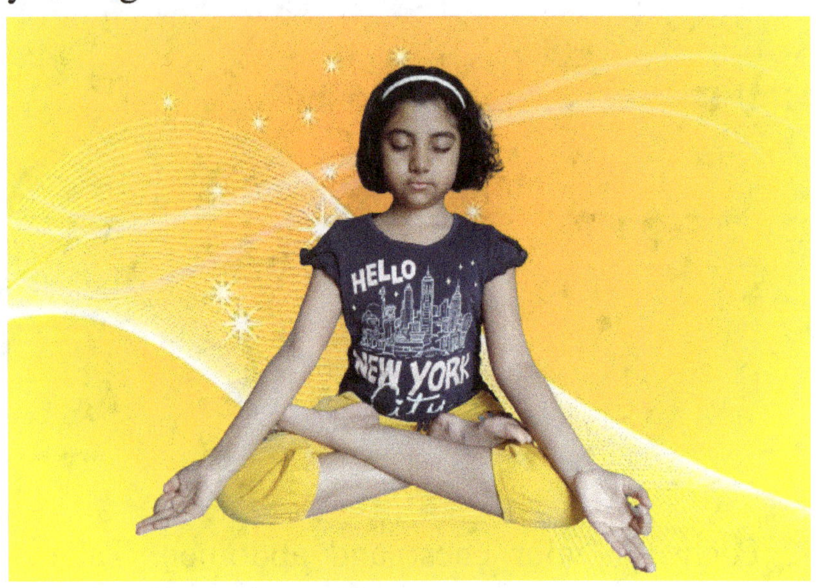

10. Finally, take a few moments to scan your entire body. If you notice any remaining tension, send your breath to that area and consciously release it.

11. Stay in this state of deep relaxation for as long as you like, allowing your mind and body to rejuvenate.

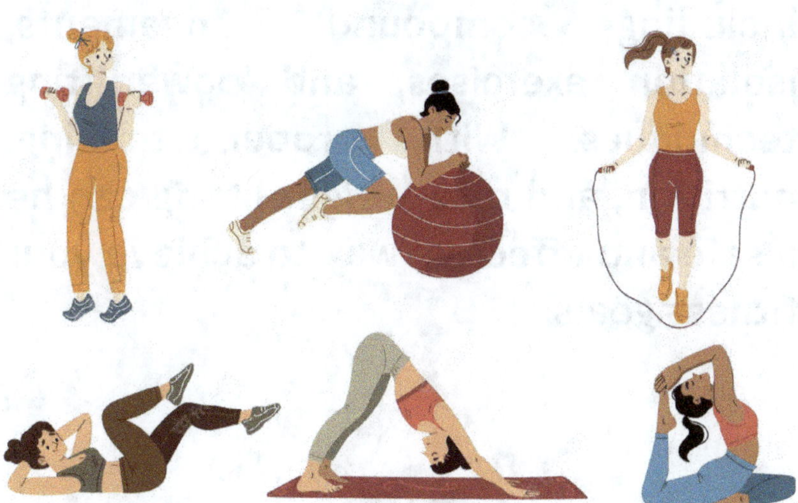

Weight lifting is a form of exercise that involves lifting weights (dumbbells, barbells, machines, etc.) to build muscle strength and endurance. It's popular among athletes, bodybuilders, and fitness enthusiasts who aim to increase their muscle mass, improve their athletic performance, and enhance their overall health. Weight lifting exercises can target specific muscles or muscle groups, such as the chest, arms, legs, back, and shoulders.

including compound movements, isolation exercises, and powerlifting techniques. With proper training, nutrition, and rest, weight lifting can be a safe and effective way to achieve your fitness goals.

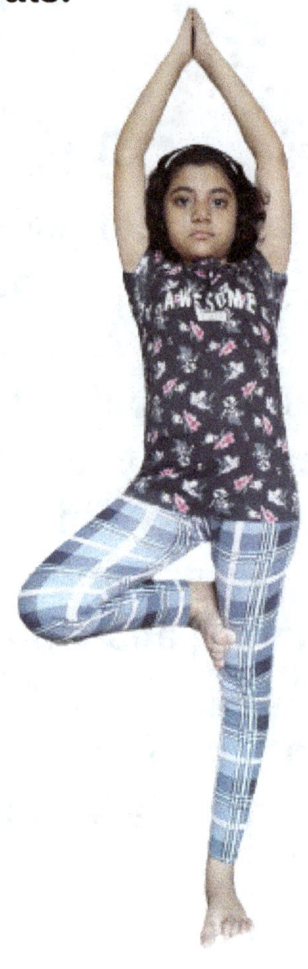

1. Improved Strength and Muscle Mass: The primary benefit of weight lifting exercise is the increase in strength and muscle mass. This is accomplished by lifting weights that are challenging, which causes the muscles to gradually increase in size and strength.

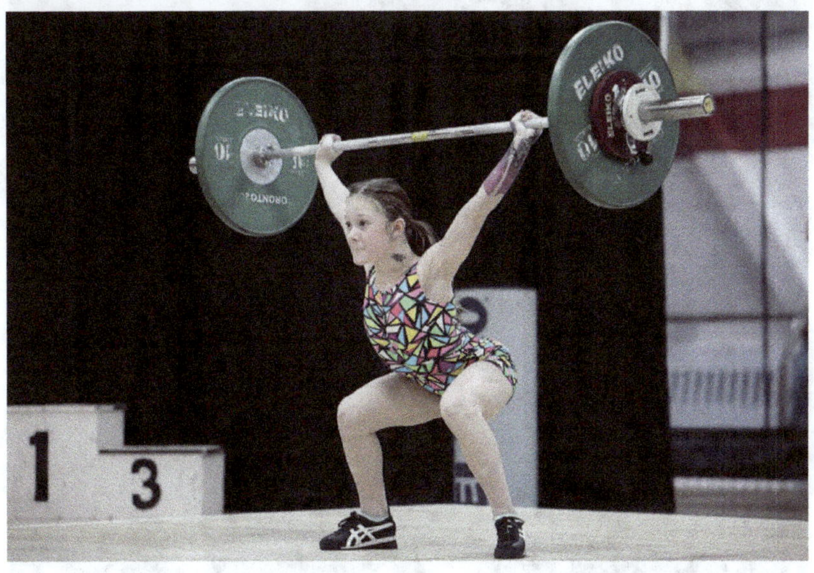

2. Improved Bone Density: Weight lifting exercise also improves bone density, which is important for preventing osteoporosis and other bone disorders. By lifting weights, the bone is put under stress, which causes it to increase in density.

3. Improved Metabolism: Weight lifting exercise also helps improve metabolism by increasing muscle mass. More muscle mass means a higher resting metabolic rate, which means that the body burns more calories at rest.

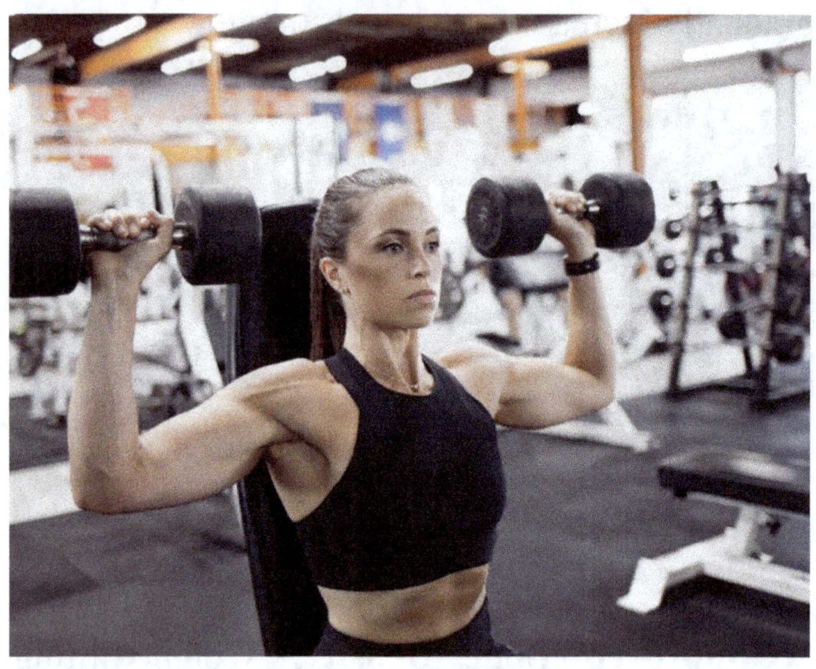

4. Decreased Risk of Injury: Weight lifting exercise can also help decrease the risk of injury by strengthening the muscles. Stronger muscles can better support the joints and help prevent injury.

Risks of Weight Lifting Exercise:

1. Injury: The primary risk of weight lifting exercise is injury, especially if it is not done properly. Common injuries include strains, sprains, and fractures.

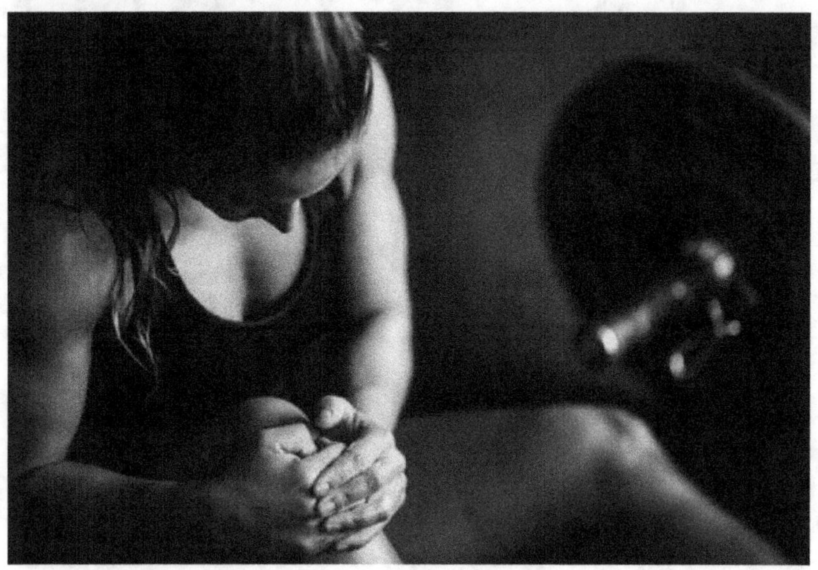

2. Muscle Soreness: Weight lifting exercise can also cause muscle soreness, especially if the exercise is new to the individual.

3. Overtraining: Weight lifting exercise can also lead to overtraining, which can cause fatigue, decreased performance, and injury.

4. Poor Technique: Poor technique can also lead to injury or decreased performance. Proper technique must be used to avoid injury and to achieve maximum benefit.

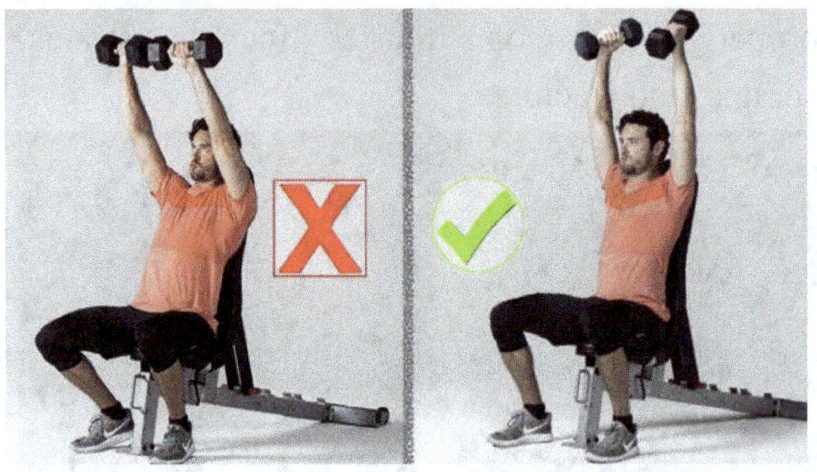

How to do Weight Lifting Exercise Properly:

1. Warm-up: It is important to warm up before starting weight lifting exercise. This can include stretching, light cardio, or other warm-up exercises.

2. Proper Technique: Using proper technique is critical in weight lifting exercise. This includes maintaining proper form, lifting with the legs and not the back, and using a spotter when necessary.

3. Gradual Progression: Gradual progression is important in weight lifting exercise. This means increasing weight or resistance gradually over time to avoid injury and to achieve maximum benefit.

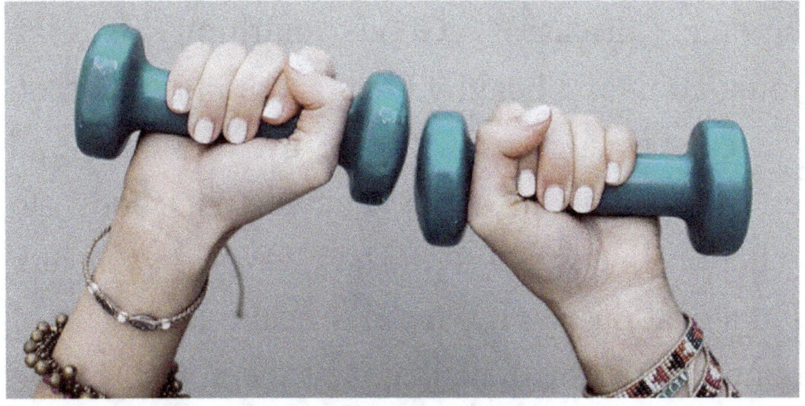

4. Adequate Rest and Recovery: Adequate rest and recovery are also critical in weight lifting exercise. This means taking breaks between sets, allowing for adequate recovery time between workouts, and getting enough sleep.

5. Proper Nutrition: Proper nutrition is also important in weight lifting exercise. This includes eating a balanced diet with adequate protein, carbohydrates, and fats to support muscle growth and recovery.

Nutrition is the study of nutrients in food, how the body uses them, and the relationship between diet, health, and disease. Health nutrition is vital for good health; it plays an essential role in maintaining optimal health and preventing chronic diseases. Good nutrition is the foundation of a healthy body and mind. The food we eat provides us with energy, nutrients, and essential minerals that enable our body to function correctly. The World Health Organization (WHO) defines health as a state of complete physical, mental, and social well-being, and not merely the absence of disease or infirmity.

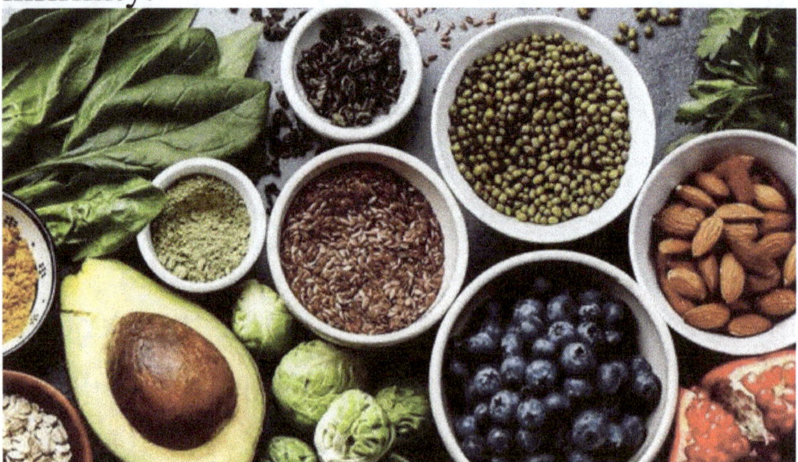

Nutrition and Growth:

Good nutrition is essential for growth and development. Nutrients such as protein, vitamins, and minerals are crucial for the proper functioning of the body. Children and teenagers require adequate nutrition for the growth and development of bones, muscles, and organs. Inadequate nutrition can lead to growth retardation, stunting, and malnutrition. A balanced diet that contains all the essential nutrients can provide the necessary energy and nutrients to support growth and development.

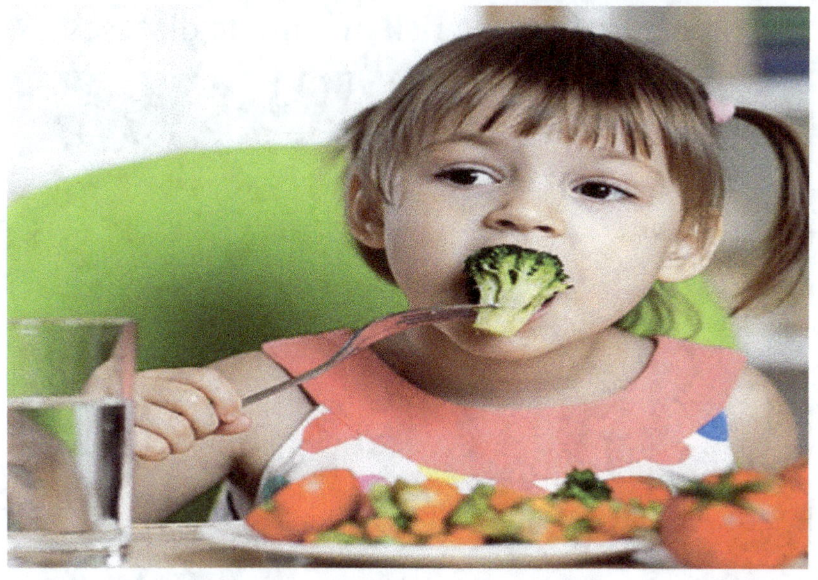

Nutrition and Disease Prevention:

A balanced diet is essential for the prevention of chronic diseases. Chronic diseases such as obesity, diabetes, heart disease, and cancer are strongly associated with a poor diet. A diet that is high in fat, sugar, and calories can lead to obesity, which is a significant risk factor for many chronic diseases. A diet that is low in fiber, vitamins, and minerals can lead to an increased risk of chronic diseases such as heart disease, cancer, and diabetes. A balanced diet that is high in fruits, vegetables, whole grains, and lean protein can reduce the risk of chronic diseases.

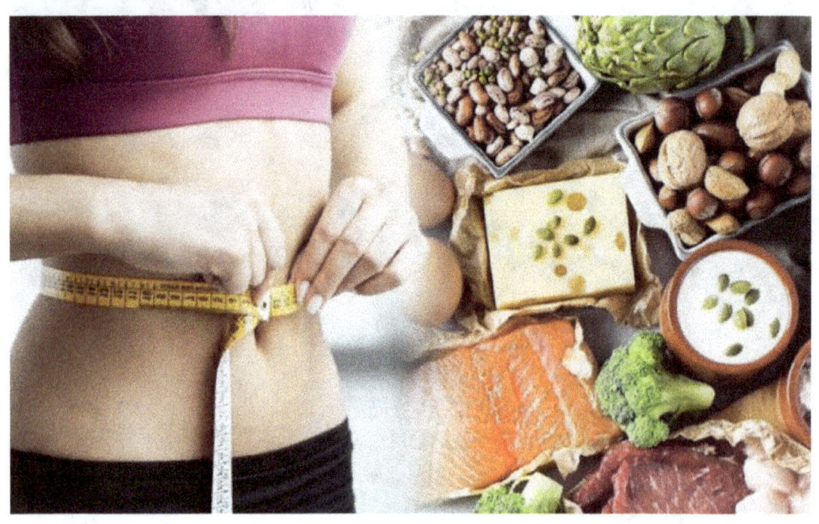

Nutrition and Mental Health:

Good nutrition is essential for mental health. Several studies have shown that a diet that is high in vegetables, fruits, whole grains, and lean protein can reduce the risk of depression and anxiety. A diet that is high in processed foods, sugar, and fat can lead to inflammation in the body and increased risk of depression and anxiety.

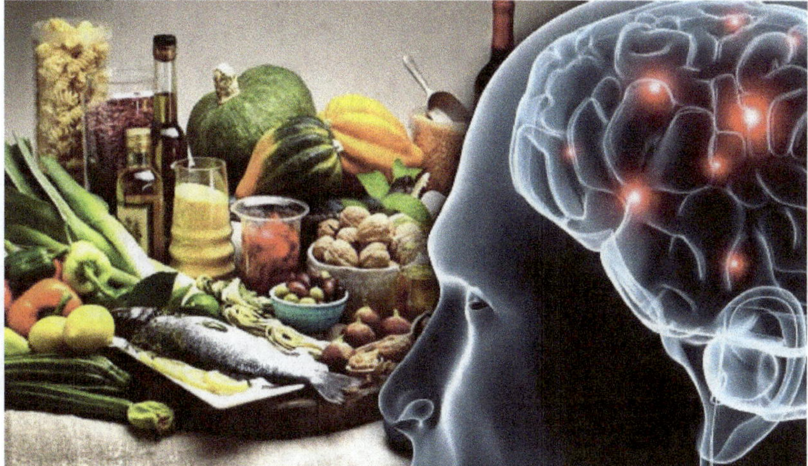

Nutrition and Immune System:

Good nutrition is essential for a healthy immune system. Nutrients such as vitamin C, D, and E, zinc, and selenium, are essential for the proper functioning of the immune system.

A diet that is high in processed foods, sugar, and refined carbohydrates can weaken the immune system and increase the risk of infections and diseases.

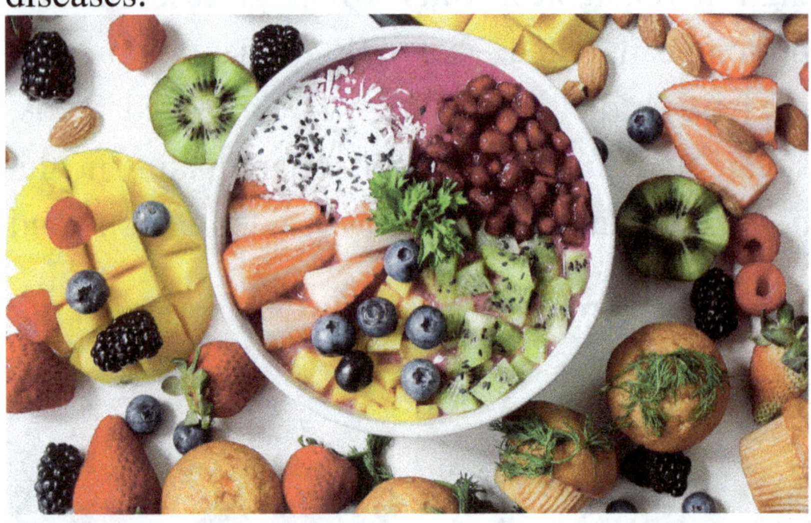

Nutrition and Aging:

Good nutrition is essential for healthy aging. As we age, our body's nutritional needs change. The need for protein, vitamins, and minerals increases, while the need for calories decreases. A diet that is high in whole grains, fruits, vegetables, and lean protein can provide the necessary nutrients to support healthy aging and prevent age-related diseases.

Nutrition and Pregnancy:

Good nutrition is essential for a healthy pregnancy. Pregnant women require adequate nutrition for the development of the fetus. Nutrients such as folic acid, iron, and calcium are essential for the healthy development of the fetus. A diet that is high in fruits, vegetables, whole grains, and lean protein can provide the necessary nutrients to support a healthy pregnancy.

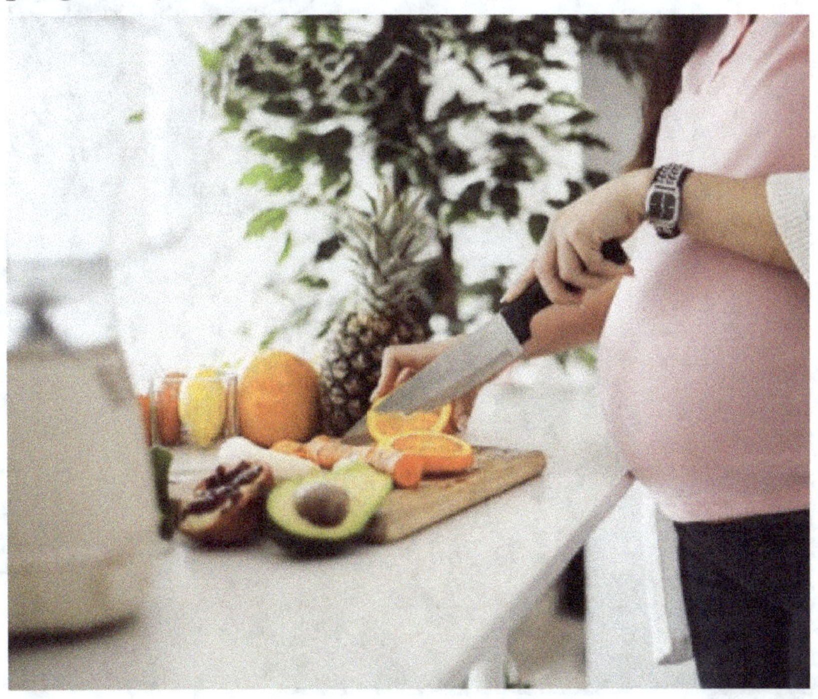

Nutrition and Breastfeeding:

Good nutrition is essential for breastfeeding mothers. Breastfeeding mothers require adequate nutrition for the production of milk and the growth of the baby. Nutrients such as protein, calcium, and iron are essential for breastfeeding mothers. A diet that is high in fruits, vegetables, whole grains, and lean protein can provide the necessary nutrients to support breastfeeding.

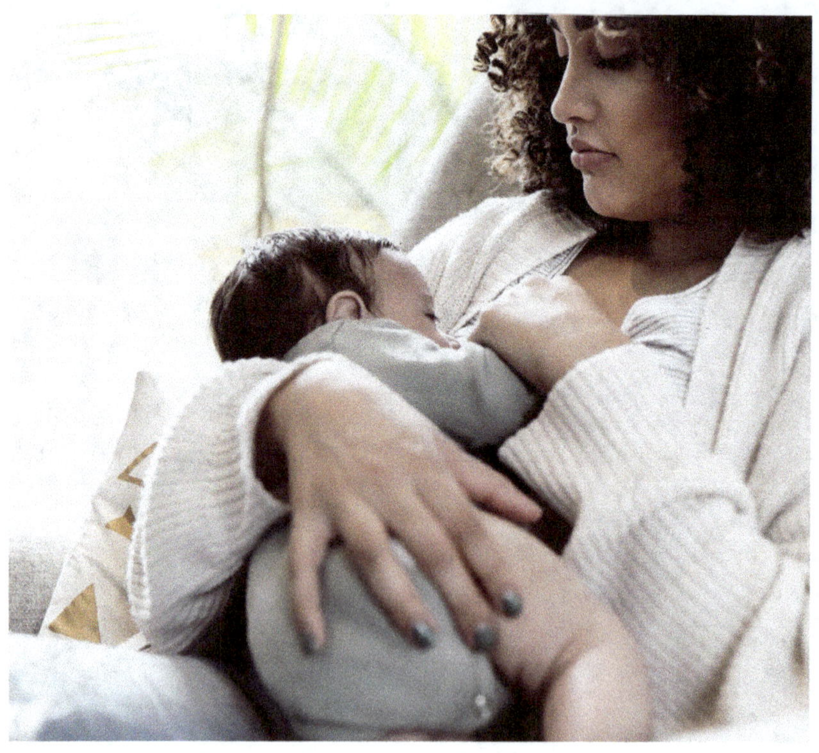

Nutrients in Healthy Foods

Unhealthy foods that we consume are usually high in fat, calories, and sugar, which makes us consume more than we require and stores excesses as fat in the body. This, in turn, increases the risk of life-threatening diseases such as obesity, diabetes, and hypertension. On the other hand, healthy foods contain all the necessary nutrients such as vitamins, minerals, and fiber, which are vital for optimal health and wellbeing.

Carbohydrates

Carbohydrates are essential for the body as they provide energy and help to maintain a good level of glucose in the blood. Eating healthy carbs from whole grains such as whole wheat, brown rice, and quinoa help to keep the body full for longer, reducing the chances of overeating.

Protein

Proteins are the building blocks of the body and are essential for proper growth and development. Eating healthy protein sources such as fish, lean meats, beans, and nuts can help keep the body functioning properly, build and repair muscles, and boost the immune system.

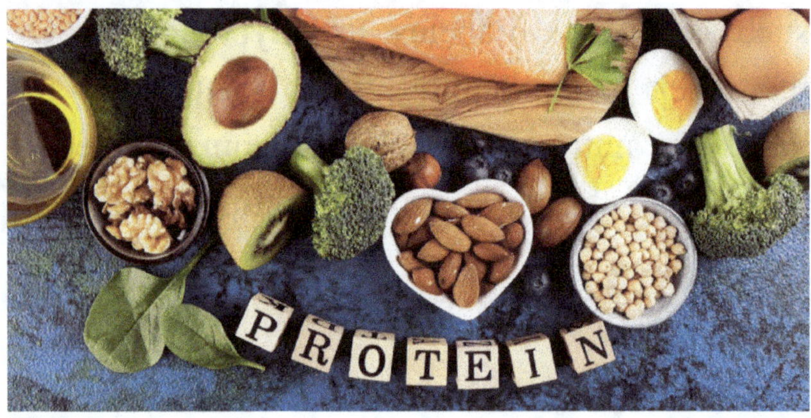

Fats

Healthy fats such as monounsaturated and polyunsaturated fats are essential for the proper functioning of the body and must be consumed in small quantities. Eating nuts, fish, and oils from plants such as olive oil can help maintain healthy cholesterol levels and reduce the risk of heart disease.

Fiber

Fiber is important for the digestive system as it helps to move waste out of the body and reduces constipation. Healthy foods such as fruits, vegetables, and whole grains are rich in fiber and keep the digestive system functioning properly.

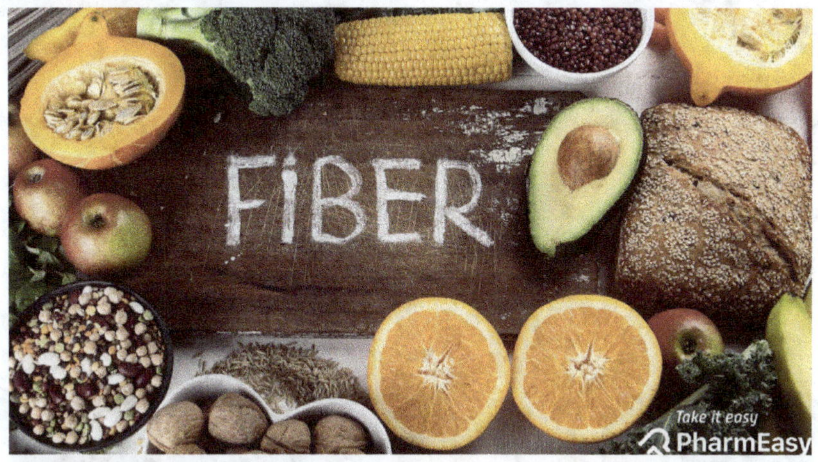

Vitamins

Healthy foods provide an excellent source of vitamins that help keep the body healthy. These vitamins include vitamins A, B, C, D, E, and K and are essential for the smooth running of the body. These vitamins perform various functions, such as keeping the skin healthy, maintaining the immune system, and strengthening bones.

Minerals

Minerals such as iron, calcium, and magnesium are essential for the proper functioning of the body. They help to build strong bones, maintain a healthy heart, and regulate the production of hormones. Foods such as dairy, dark green leafy vegetables, nuts, and seeds are good sources of minerals.

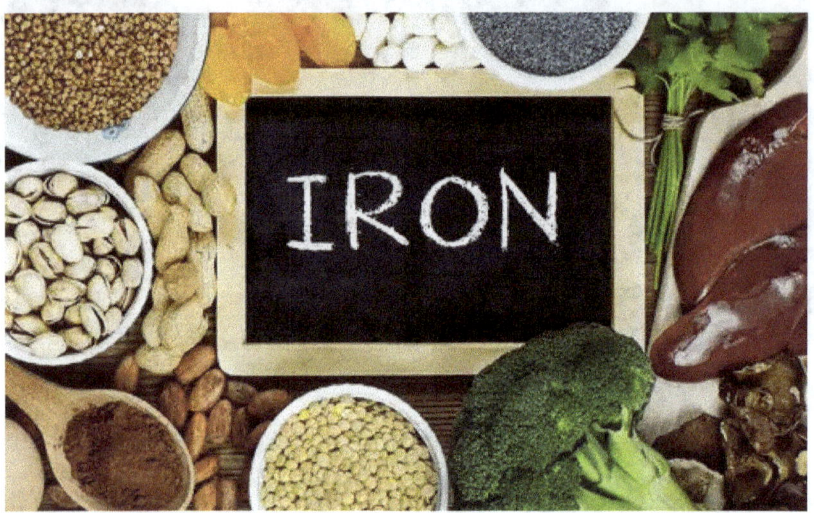

Importance of Healthy Eating

Healthy eating is important for several reasons. The following are some of the major reasons why we should all make healthy food choices:

Heart Health

Eating a diet rich in fruits, vegetables, and whole grains can help to lower blood pressure, cholesterol levels, and reduce the risk of heart disease. Healthy fats such as omega-3 fatty acids in fish also help to lower the risk of heart diseases.

8 Amazing Heart Healthy Foods

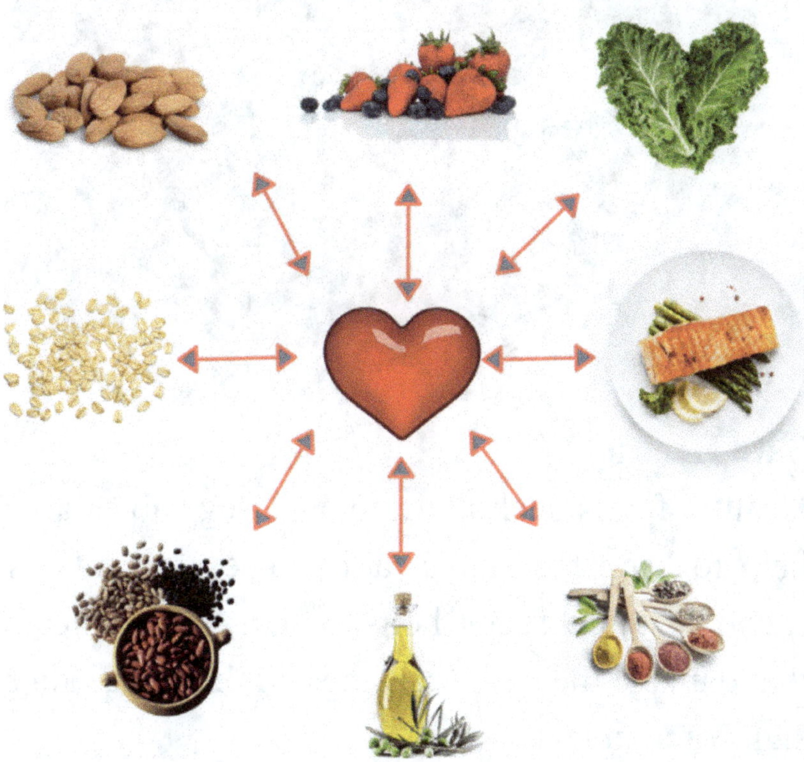

Weight Control

Eating healthy food and limiting high-calorie foods can help control weight, reducing the risk of obesity and related diseases.

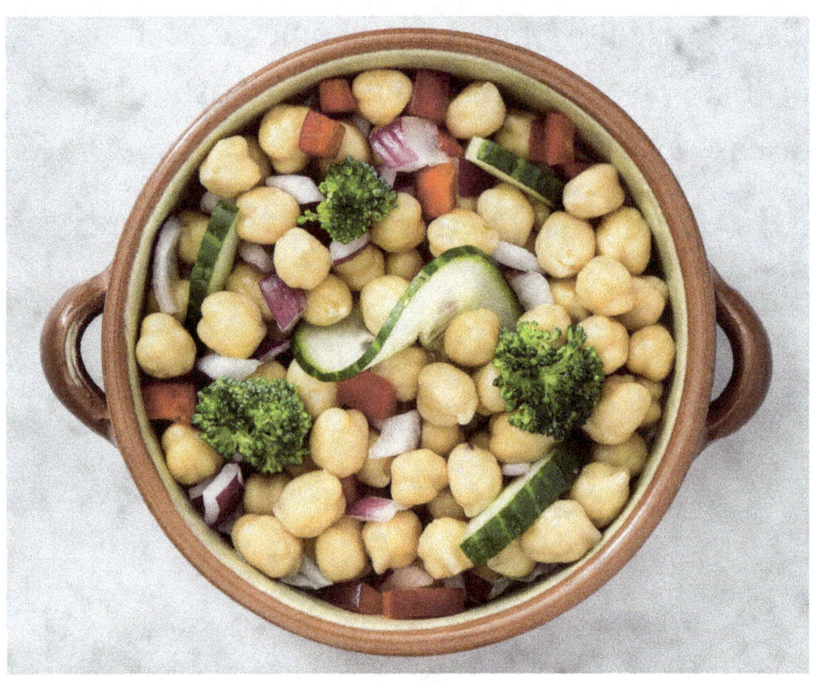

Skin Health

Healthy foods such as fruits and vegetables also help to keep the skin healthy. The antioxidants found in these foods help to fight free radicals that damage the cells, causing wrinkles and other signs of aging.

Improved Brain Health

Healthy food is essential for maintaining brain health and reducing the risk of cognitive decline. Nutrients found in healthy foods such as omega-3 fatty acids are vital for maintaining healthy brain function, preventing memory loss, and reducing the risk of diseases such as Alzheimer's.

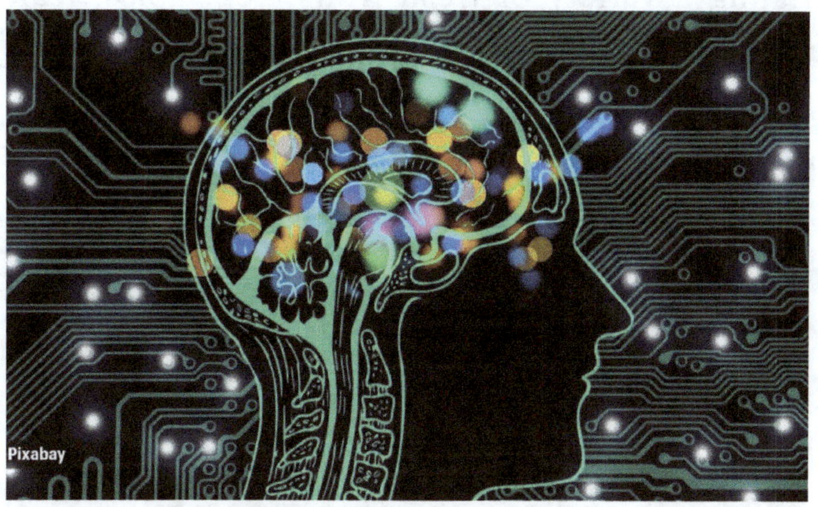

Reduced Stress Levels

Eating healthy food and exercising can help reduce stress levels, thereby reducing the risk of stress-related conditions such as depression, anxiety, and high blood pressure.

How to Eat Healthy

The following are some tips on how to eat healthy:

Eat a Balanced Diet

Eating a balanced diet that contains all the necessary nutrients is essential for good health. Eating a variety of fresh fruits, vegetables, lean meats, nuts, and whole grains can help the body get all the nutrients it needs.

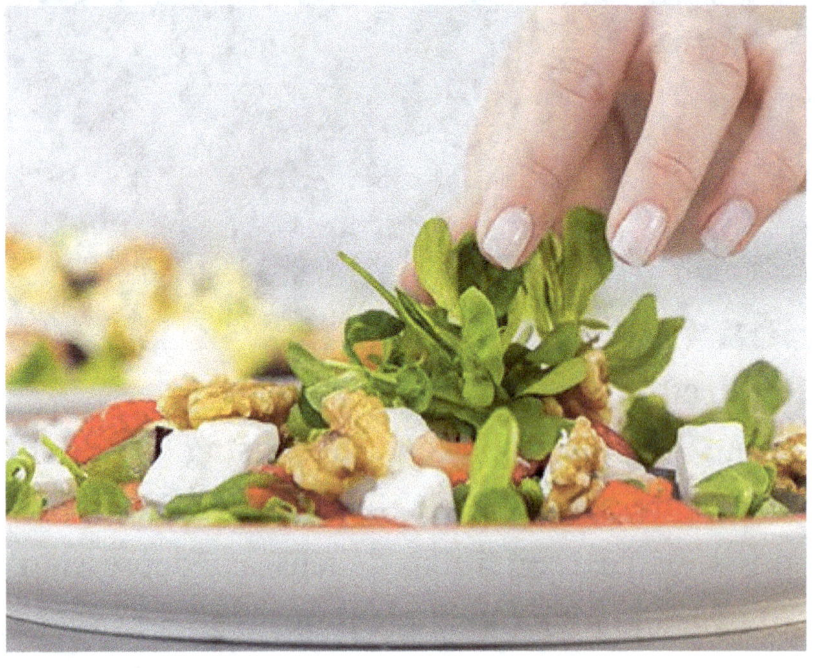

Limit Sugar and Salt

Limiting the intake of sugar and salt is essential for maintaining good health. High intake of sugar and salt can lead to several diseases, including high blood pressure, diabetes, and obesity.

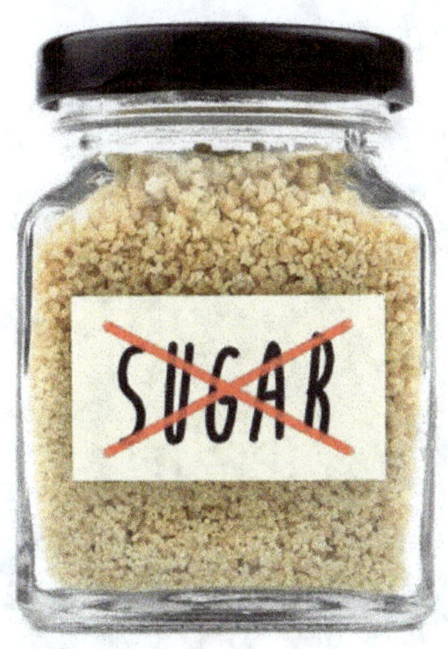

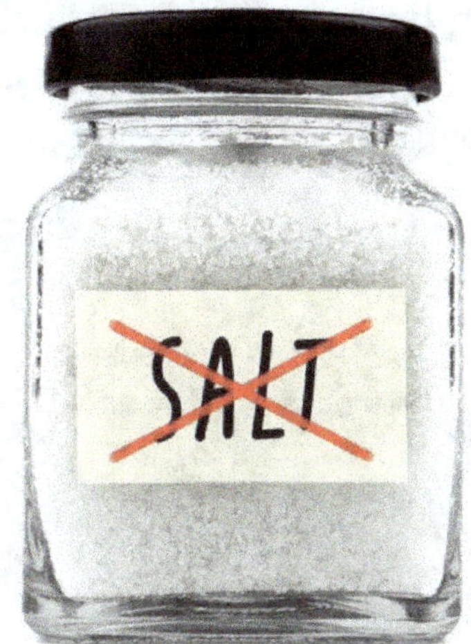

Stay Hydrated

Drinking plenty of water keeps the body hydrated and functioning properly. Drinking water also helps to flush out toxins and waste from the body.

Avoid Processed Foods

Processed foods contain sugar, added fats, and high levels of salt, which can lead to weight gain, inflammation, and an increased risk of chronic conditions. Limiting the intake of processed foods and opting for fresh fruits and vegetables can help maintain good health.

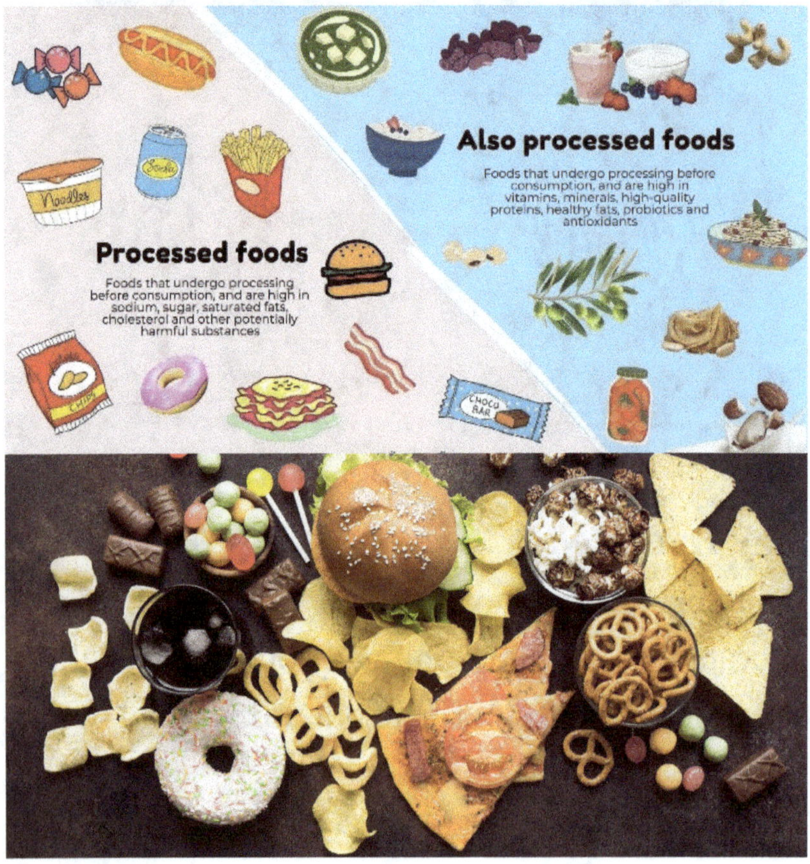

Fasting has been studied extensively, with research showing that it can have numerous health benefits for the human body. It can regulate blood sugar levels, boost the immune system, decrease inflammation, and improve metabolic health. Fasting has also been linked to improvements in brain function and an increase in lifespan

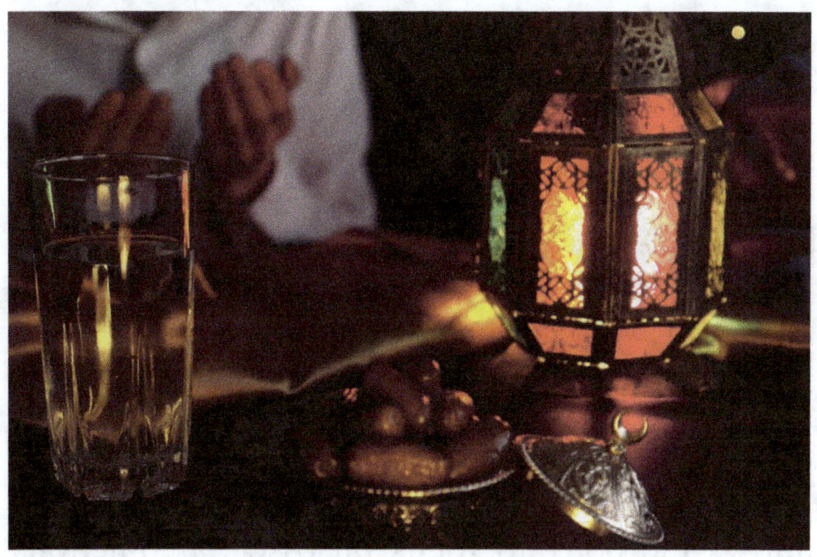

Fasting is a highly versatile practice, with various types of fasting available to individuals depending on their preferences and goals. The following are some popular types of fasting:

1. Weight Loss: Fasting can lead to weight loss due to decreased calorie intake. When the body is in a state of fasting, it uses its fat stores for energy, which can lead to weight loss over time.

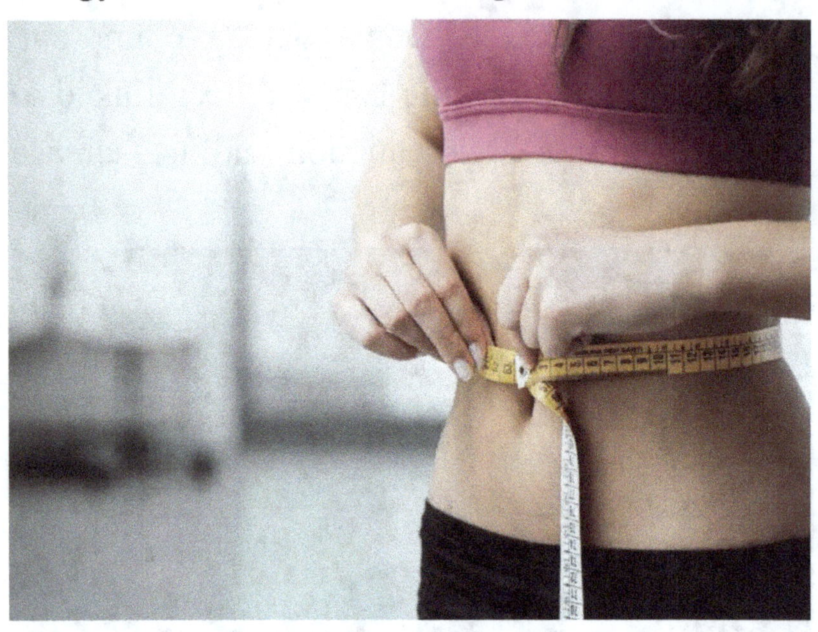

2. Improved Mental Clarity: Fasting can improve mental clarity as it eliminates sugar and allows the body to focus on essential functions such as detoxification, cellular repair, and immune function. A clear mind can help individuals make better decisions, improve productivity, and reduce stress.

3. Reduced Inflammation: Fasting can lead to reduced inflammation in the body, which can lead to a lower risk of developing chronic diseases such as diabetes, cancer, and heart disease.

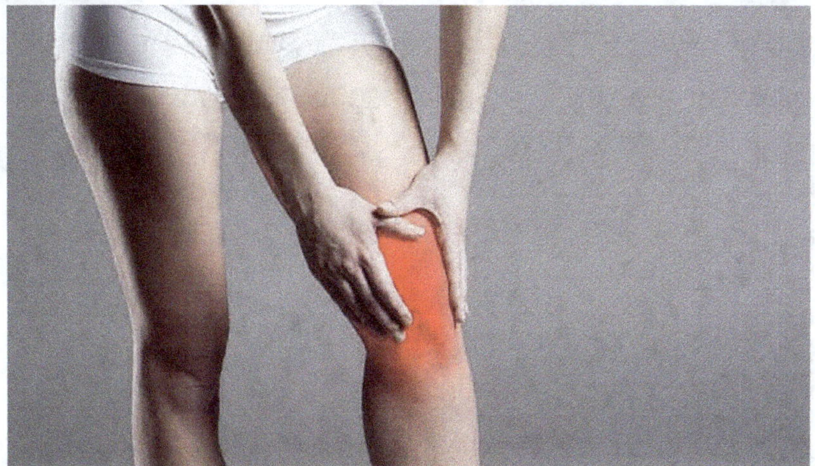

4. Improved Immune System: Fasting can lead to an improvement in the immune system, as it allows the body to focus on detoxification and cellular repair.

5. Improved Metabolic Health: Fasting has been shown to improve metabolic health, including the reduction of insulin resistance, lower blood sugar levels, and decrease the risk of developing type 2 diabetes.

Social Support Networks

Finally, having a strong social support network can also have a positive impact on your mental health. Surrounding yourself with positive, supportive people can help to reduce feelings of stress, anxiety, and depression, while also providing a sense of purpose and belonging.

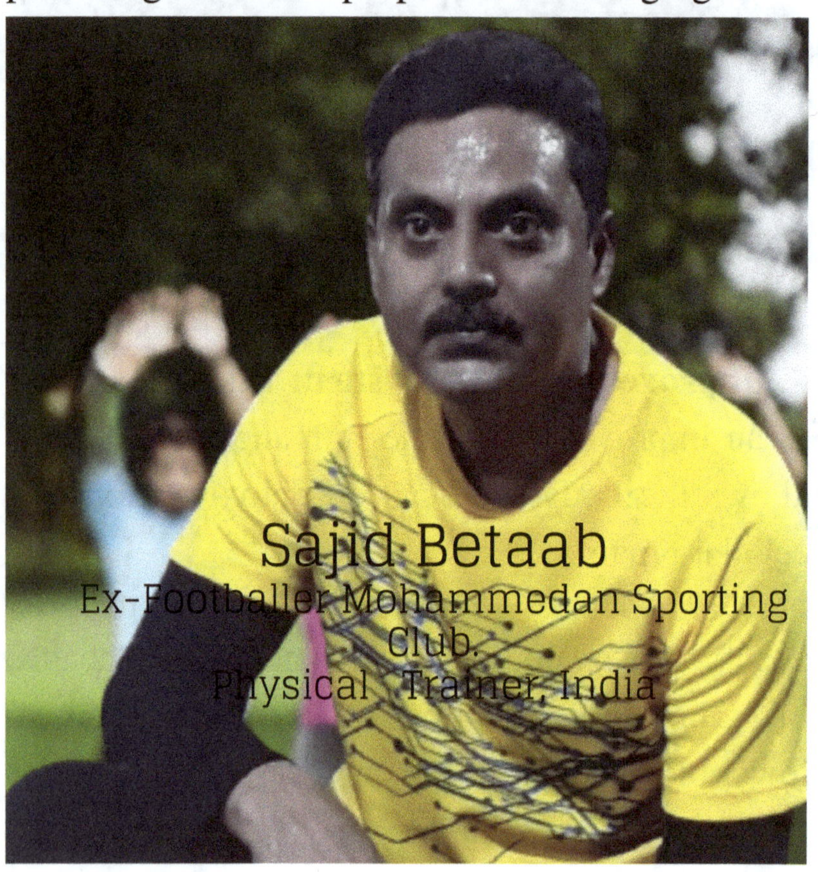